YOU ARE NOT THE MAN YOU
ARE SUPPOSED TO BE

You Are Not the Man You Are Supposed to Be

Into the Chaos of Modern Masculinity

MARTIN ROBINSON

BLOOMSBURY CONTINUUM
LONDON · OXFORD · NEW YORK · NEW DELHI · SYDNEY

BLOOMSBURY CONTINUUM
Bloomsbury Publishing Plc
50 Bedford Square, London, WC1B 3DP, UK
29 Earlsfort Terrace, Dublin 2, Ireland

BLOOMSBURY, BLOOMSBURY CONTINUUM and the Diana logo are trademarks
of Bloomsbury Publishing Plc

First published in Great Britain 2021

A catalogue record for this book is available from the British Library

ISBN: HB: 978-1-4729-7127-2; eBook: 978-1-4729-7128-9; ePDF: 978-1-4729-7125-8

2 4 6 8 10 9 7 5 3 1

Typeset by Deanta Global Publishing Services, Chennai, India
Printed and bound in Great Britain by CPI Group (UK) Ltd, Croydon CR0 4YY

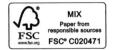

To find out more about our authors and books visit www.bloomsbury.com
and sign up for our newsletters

For Marian, and our children

Contents

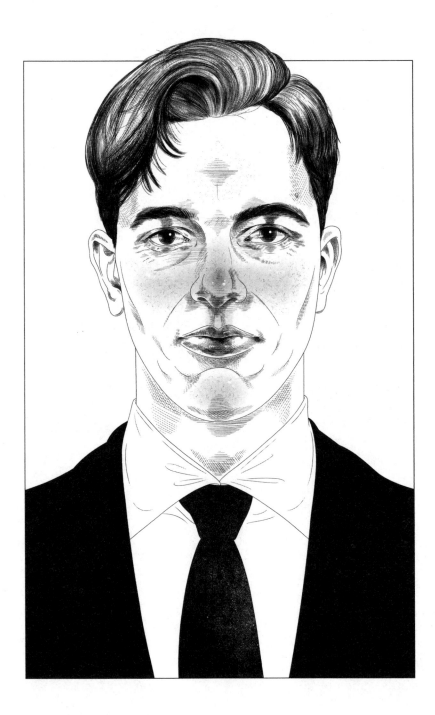

Prologue

I am a man. At least, that's the assumption I'd been working with. Paperwork would certainly concur – any registration form or doctor's file or police report: 'Man'. Who was I to argue with admin?

Having the good fortune of maleness meant I wasn't supposed to be afraid, but in my usual anarchic manner I was pushing the boundaries, with a daring bout of fear electrified by some dazzling weakness.

The fear was not new. Quite honestly, I'm afraid all the time: of muggings, terrorism, cancer (bone the current favourite), spreadsheets, sweaty handshakes, home intruders, stilted conversations, getting nutmegged at football by my children, falling safes – on it goes . . . Right now, though, I found myself stung by my fear of all fears: a fear worse even than death. Exposure. I am a fiercely private person. Not out of high-mindedness, or a grand moral response to the circlejerk of social media, but simply for self-protection. *Can't let anyone see the rot inside here.* I'll do anything to avoid revealing too much about myself, including ironic deflection, playing dumb, feigning sleep and hiding behind large items of furniture.

'What is *The Book of Man*?'

My right hand, I noticed, was shaking from last night's whisky binge, so I hid it under the table with my left. When I spoke, the words came out fast and giddy, in a way so out of character it could only mean I was still drunk. The risk of betraying myself was very real.

The Book of Man *is a new digital men's magazine which aims to look at men's inner lives rather than the outward display. I'm a journalist who's worked in men's magazines for my entire career, and I founded* The Book of Man *to do something different. To look at issues like mental health and masculinity rather than expensive suits and diving watches. It's supposed to be a supportive look behind the curtain of the male psyche.*

The microphone at my dry lips was a fat sponge soaking it all up. Opposite me was the podcast host, Lucy Donoughue from *Happiful* magazine, who was soothing, trustworthy and empathetic: exactly what I didn't need if I was going to get through this without spilling everything.

'Tell us about the New Masculinity,' she said.

The New Masculinity is about questioning the old-school ways of being a man, and suggesting new ideals such as empathy, kindness, emotional strength, honesty, vulnerability. It's not about telling men off: it's a vision of expansion.

'What does being a father mean to you?'

It's the purpose I've been searching for my whole life. I think I was very unhappy and self-destructive before, but now I need to see beyond myself to my children's lives, their future.

'What have been your experiences with depression?'

That's it. Pull the ripcord, break glass for emergency, signal for a substitution. The question was in the pre-agreed notes, but my usual attention to detail – i.e. a glance while thumbing through Instagram – had once again landed me out of my depth. For all my messaging about how important it is for men to open up about their issues, I'd never talked about mine. Years had been spent building up a protective shell in the general shape of an adult male, which I wasn't about to slither out of just to have the courage of my convictions. Shame my mouth had decided to have its yearly stretch, yammering away like some hopped-up nightclub compère raised from the dead.

I've never really opened up about this before. It's been lifelong, I think. For me it manifested itself in silence. I was a virtual mute for a great deal of my life, pretty much unable to speak in the company of others. It always felt like I had this wall in my head which I couldn't get through. It still occasionally comes back even now . . .

I tucked my hands under my thighs.

'Last question: what would you say to your teenage self?'

Inside my head a VHS tape was inserted into a top-loading player. On the screen the old tape took a few seconds to catch, but then I saw myself sat on the floor of my bedroom, listening to Nirvana's *In Utero* on my CD Walkman, wearing a Joy Division T-shirt, with photos of Marlon Brando and Beatrice Dalle taped to the wall. Trying to absorb dark materials to bring an existential glamour to my typical teenage problems of bad skin, extreme embarrassment and a conviction that my life was already over. It was in moments like these that I was subconsciously constructing that adult shell, while shutting away the vulnerable child left inside.

I'd say to myself: get a haircut. Buy some decent clothes. And . . . it'll be OK.

And that's when I cried. Not a solitary Gregory Peck tear either, but a facial explosion of goop. Hot waves of rabid sobs couldn't be stemmed, no matter how deeply I plunged my face into the crook of my arm. *It's the whisky, it's the whisky,* I gasped into the mic, before Lucy gently ended the show.

What a disaster. What a betrayal of myself. As sometimes happens when your worst nightmare becomes reality, I had a rush of mortified exhilaration and found myself alternating between crying and laughing, until they became one, contorting my face into an expression only usually spotted on church gargoyles or in 1970s pornography. I hugged Lucy, stumbled out of the booth, apologized to everyone and got out onto the street.

Dizzied, I walked around the block, accidentally jostling the lunchtime Fitzrovia crowd as I looked for air. Some of the men pushed back, their hard bodies forming walls around me; not men in a city but a city made of men. In their glare I was ashamed to be seen crying like this. Exposed as not one of them.

A pub appeared, a sticky-floored womb for broken man-babies. I went in, ordered a pie and a pint, sat down at a table, wiped at my eyes, and thumbed at my phone. Within a minute the pint was half gone and I wasn't crying any more. That's all it takes to repair the front. Before I was completely together again there was time to ponder the disappearing cracks. If I prised them apart what would I find? The secrets to my soul – or nothing at all?

Am I normal?

The question had always chewed on me. A recent addition was: could I be diagnosed with a mental health disorder? It was likely there'd be one that fitted my symptoms, but it was too late, I felt: my dysfunction had been exacerbated beyond repair because I'd never faced up to it. It's not what men do. We bury the worst and carry on, pretending not to hear the scratching beneath the soil.

I drained the drink, bought another. Thumbed at my phone again, put it down.

I'm not a man. Not the man I'm supposed to be.

I was spending my days reporting on men while avoiding a hard look at myself. For too many years I'd followed an idea of what a man is; one I had come to loathe, but never escape – there was an inevitability about it. In my younger days, I'd simply allowed myself to be battered into man shape by life as it presented itself. Dutifully I'd accepted the herding from school to university to work, picking up lessons in manliness from whoever was drinking opposite me. The closest I'd come to an individualistic code of living was half-remembered dialogue from kung-fu movies. Drifting in this way your concern can be about fitting in rather than making decisions for yourself. You have no clue as to what you want, or what might bring personal fulfilment: instead you follow what's around you and hope to stumble into a lifestyle that isn't too depressing. As for applying intellect, forget it: lost mine at Reading Festival in 2006. The thing is, though, if you're a man from a middle-class background – lower middle-class in my case (he says, a little too quickly) – you can drift and do well in life, just as upper-class men can drift into running the country, and working-class men can drift right out of existence.

In *The Descent of Man* Grayson Perry called white, middle-class, middle-aged men the 'zero longitude of identity' against which everything is judged. The behaviours that make up this identity are, he wrote, so omnipresent as, paradoxically, to make masculinity 'invisible', with the result that trying to speak to such men about it is 'like talking to a fish about water'. We don't really see what every other gender is complaining about because we don't even recognize masculinity as a type of behaviour. '*This is just the way people do things, isn't it?*'

In truth, it wasn't mere lazy acquiescence on my part, but involved a secret desperation. The desire for this invisibility has guided my life for a long time. Having always felt different, all I wanted was to match the masculinity around me and disappear inside its cloak. When you feel a freak you are desperate to be ordinary. Was it just me driven in this way, then, or was a similar urge at play even for your swaggering Alpha broskis? After all, we have to learn how to navigate our environments, and to learn you imitate. When positions of power are seen to be occupied by a certain zero-longitudinal type of man, it makes sense to conform to that model without questioning it. But should your life be a sleepwalk down a well-worn path? More pertinently: who is being trampled on as men lead their Normal Lives?

In recent times tin buckets have been thrown at our heads to wake us up. If men have been operating on the maxim that 'If it ain't broke, don't fix it,' then 'it' is now clearly falling apart, and we can no longer pretend it isn't. We have been forced to look at ourselves by a rising tide of gender equality whose diverse voices now demand rights and respect denied them by a men-first world. Grayson Perry was echoing Simone de Beauvoir's view that men are judged as the standard human being, with women thereby viewed as less than human. This 'default male' has been identified as the bogeyman, his privileged existence based upon the oppression of women, People of Colour, diverse sexualities, anyone who is 'different'. The evidence for all this is hard to deny, since it is, y'know, the history of Western religion, tradition and imperialism, but many men still try their hardest. Even those with a conscience have lapsed into a guilty silence, thinking, 'Best just hang back here for a while . . .'

Yet it's vital to engage with this, especially because the world we have presided over is no longer beneficial for the wellbeing of most men either, if it ever was. Suicide is the biggest killer in the UK of men under 45. In recent years it has been the orange flare in the night sky, illuminating a heaving ocean of self-harm, addiction, eating disorders, violence and anti-social behaviour. 95 per cent of prisoners are male, 86 per cent of homeless people, 73 per cent of deaths from drug misuse. Questioning the way we are may be difficult for men – that it's considered 'unmanly' illustrates the bind we're in – but for the good of everyone there is an urgent requirement to.

By now I was wasted. My happy-unhappy place, hollowed out but held in man-shape by booze. Whatever our experience and upbringing, sooner or later, it seemed to me, we all find ourselves in the same place: staring blankly at oblivion in a glass while the false front crumbles. But I couldn't even trust that conclusion. This entire scene, of tears falling into a pint, was a cliché of male despair. Was it even real – or was I just behaving in the way I thought men did at such moments?

No doubt much of the unhappiness in men, and caused by men, is a result of us *acting out* manliness: performing to expectations and trying to live up to the illusion. In doing so we exert a tyranny over not just others but ourselves, denying how we truly feel, what we truly want and when we need help. It means that to be a 'man' is to live a lie.

My life was ostensibly pretty successful, but the person I'd become didn't feel right, like a copy of a copy of someone else's dream. To cope, I'd taught myself not to feel. Yet the pain and sorrow remained, clearly, ready to bust out and destroy my veneer of control at the merest probing. Wasn't it time to pull apart what makes us men – to find some answers for myself in the chaos, and perhaps for others too? Not self-help: more like self-resuscitation. We needed a new way to live.

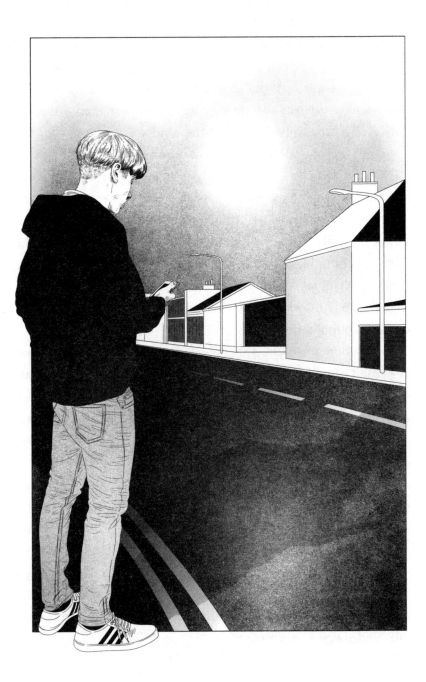

1

You Are In Control

Mental Health and Masculinity

Welcome to Hell.

Sorry, my mistake.

Welcome to Hull.

It was six months before the virus hit, when social distancing was a failure of nerve, not an act of survival. I was standing behind steel railings on an industrial estate, watching the Humber estuary beyond the dual carriageway continuing its duty of flushing away a quarter of England's effluent. Upstream the Humber Bridge sprawled doggedly across the banks. Well, Philip Larkin seemed to be inspired by the view. Mind you, so were Throbbing Gristle.

Hull – Hell? Hilarious. No-one here has heard that before. That's the last joke I'll make about this long-suffering place where the last major improvement in the standard of living was adding chicken spice to takeaway chips. No, I won't judge Hull as others do, as a degraded expanse of collapsed industry stinking of cod and heroin; not when my neglected family are from here. I know my roots, and I'm always loyal enough to protest whenever it's voted the UK's crappest town: 'It's a city, OK?'

I walked on.

'In one hundred yards, turn right.'

Smartphones aren't smart enough to detect regret about where you're headed, or the masochism that instructed it in the first place. I started thumbing through Instagram memes.

That one mate who can't grow a beard/
@TheRock: 'Let's get the blood flowin'/
REAL Men Starve Their Flesh And Feed Their Spirit /
Your Hustle Is More Important Than Pussy/

I looked up. Old-school reality was everywhere. The September evening sunshine brought a warm glow to the rented units, barbed wire and burned-out cars, as though God had downed a can of Strongbow and suddenly felt far fonder of his piss-soaked trouser of a Creation. Business signs I'd normally take no notice of seemed to vibrate with meaning.

'Hot tub specialist. "Water that moves you."'

'Tornado Gym.'

'Heavenly Services, affordable funerals, £1,700.'

A lorry thundered past: 'Bulk liquids. Feed products only.'

Maybe not that much meaning.

I turned right onto an exposed stretch of road leading to my destination. A boarded-up pub on the corner had a St George's Cross Blu-Tacked to the inside of a dirty window. England and its men: facing ruin. Individual breakdowns mirroring the national breakdown. At least we have our memories, our shared hallucinations of English history. Defeating the Jerries, the Bosh, the Armada, in whatever order, and we ruled, ruled the waves, thrashing the savages and taking the tea and sugar that was rightfully ours. Oh, remember when Henry VIII killed his wives,

Churchill won the war, we raised the World Cup, pulled off *The Italian Job* and Gazza was the only one who cried! Remember when things were better? When it was jolly old England, when it was 'En-Ger-Land, En-Ger-Land, En-Ger-Land', and when men *were* men . . .

I'm a man, or at least a decent imitation. The shell 'Martin Robinson' has been refined over the years as an effective vehicle to survive in the world with particular mannerisms and attitudes for a frictionless existence. This stooped figure was on the defensive, but instinctively working hard not to show it as he entered unknown territory where Real Men lurk. Check out his eyes-to-the-ground walk: not a victim, but not an instigator of trouble either. Existing in liminal spaces, in train vestibules or on a conversation's periphery, he's that invisibly ubiquitous being, a Default Male. The one problem this evening was the jacket.

On the other side of the street a bunch of lads were heading for the first pint of the night with the kind of shaved heads you only get in the North, where the clippers have touched bone. Defensively I zipped up my North Face waterproof, thrown on in an attempt to look less like a heavily moisturized London media wanker, but which only served to identify me as one so far up his own arse he can't even dress for the weather.

What am I doing here?

'Martin Robinson' was about to have his bloody doors blown off.

'Your destination is straight ahead.'

Down the street outside the Airco training centre a group of men in shorts raised their heads towards me. Human contact. On its heels would be vulnerability. Beyond that, potential honesty. I wanted to turn and run, but it was too late.

'Hello, mate – you looking for us?'

The men were all wearing black 'Andy's Man Club' T-shirts. I was looking for Andy's Man Club.

Yes.

'First time, is it? That's great. In this way, mate: they'll show you through . . .'

As I was led inside by a couple more big men in shorts and AMC T-shirts I ignored another first-timer beside me, a pensioner, to look at my phone for comfort, my usual recourse when I'm not being directly addressed.

'What's your name?'

Oh. It's Martin.

'You can have a brew and wait in there, Martin. Don't worry, you'll be fine.'

More big men in shorts and AMC T-shirts waited in a tea-making corner. I unzipped my waterproof, made tea with a tremulous hand and pretended I didn't spill half of it down my leg. While my jeans steamed the other men took my watering eyes for panic and began to take me under their collective wing.

'You'll be fine, you know. What's your name?'

Martin.

'It's like Fight Club here, without the fighting.'

And today you have the leeching narrator.

Andy's Man Club is a new, free, no-nonsense men's mental health support group which runs nationwide and has its biggest group here in Hull. It was set up two years ago by a former rugby player from Halifax called Luke Ambler, after the suicide of his brother-in-law. Luke wanted to provide a safe space for men to talk about their problems. Now every Monday night over a thousand men around the country come to their meetings in 28 cities. It is one of the most remarkable organizations – spread by word of mouth – in a country of men dealing with their mental health for the first time.

'I don't know why my nurse told me to come here. What's it all about?' The old guy was talking to me. I shrugged in feigned ignorance, but he pressed on, saying he was mostly stuck at home these days after a bad fall put him out of work at 70. 'It's all right, though,' he said, 'because daytime TV is so good.' I liked the sarcasm. I liked him. He told me about being a pilot, when his plane seat was moulded around his problematic back: the problems had come from boyhood: 'I remember my first day at school, and I looked down the line at the other kids, who were all way shorter than me – so I stooped to fit in. I used to be as tall as you. You should be careful.'

But hunching is my one true gift.

'Time to start, gents,' said one of the men in shorts. 'Let's split you up.'

I was sat in the circle of chairs watching the tip of my shoe bending against the carpet. We waited in silence. I sensed everyone had identified me as an imposter. Defensively, I'd kept my jacket on, despite the sun blazing in through the window, giving me a level of comfort akin to a third-division footballer trapped inside a tanning bed. The business-training-centre environment wasn't helping either. Flashbacks of staff away days: watching alpha bosses go through their routines of dominance and forced bonhomie while I sat with a wilting grin praying for an aneurysm to strike down either them or me, whichever was quickest.

The facilitator finally arrived, another easy-mannered fellow in shorts notably lacking in 'Silverback' room-ownership. He explained the format: a rugby ball would be passed round and you could only speak when you had it. Four questions would be asked, three standard:

'How's your week been?'

'Who's a positive person in your life?'

'Anything you want to get off your chest?'

– plus a wild card at the end. 'Anything you want to get off your chest?' was the big one, said the facilitator, where you could talk about what's really happening with you – but there was no pressure to answer it, or any of them.

'First question, then: How's your week been?'

The ball started its journey around the circle. The two people before me were too distressed to answer, so the ball reached me before I was ready with a deflecting answer.

My week's been good, because I've come back up home and decided to address some of my mental health issues which I have never truly faced. Being in this room is the start of a long journey for me.

Surprised by the honesty which had sneaked out, I was further taken aback when the other men warmly applauded. Still, I remained more mollusc than man.

As the session developed, with warmth and wit in the true Hull manner, one I always forget, it became clear that the condescension I'd walked in with was utterly misplaced. Here was a broad mix, from businessmen to brickies, taking the bold step of seeking help, which for a man comes as naturally as childbirth. Even more impressively, they were displaying emotional intelligence, something always viewed as a blind spot for men. Given the chance to explore their feelings, on the strict understanding that no-one would take the piss, they were free to express untapped aspects of themselves.

Stereotypes decree that men are cold, unemotional creatures. These men showed they *had* feelings: they just usually kept them hidden away. You could see this in the body language: how they unfurled from their arms-folded positions to animate their stories. One bloke bounced out of his seat as he described having his life turned around after his first visit here. Another credited it with transforming his relationship with his wife, shedding a tear when recounting the care she'd shown for him during his struggle. The mental health problems ranged from illnesses like borderline personality disorder or bipolar to relationship breakdowns, bereavement and job loss, but all were treated with equal validity. There were no answers given, and no answers required; talking it through was itself a means to gain understanding.

This kind of session would be familiar to those who've experienced Alcoholics Anonymous or similar programmes, but it's remarkable to think that AMC has applied it to an issue as commonly taboo as men's mental health with such rapid success. Truly, mental health awareness has gripped the country by the shoulders: the word is out at every level of society. The real issue being dealt with at Andy's Man Club, though, I'd argue, is being a man. The understanding is clear in the room: that men's inner lives are suppressed, leading to secret shame revealed in outward destruction. You could even call these sessions 'Masculinity Anonymous' – if you wanted to stop men from coming.

Meanwhile, my own barriers had been raised again. If the others were unfurling like flowers, I was curling up like a weed. The ball landed like a grenade in my lap bearing the question, 'Anything you want to get off your chest?'

Well, you know, I'm not quite ready to, er, talk about everything, but I think it's brilliant what you're all doing, it's seriously impressive, so respect to you all.

No applause this time, despite the elegant way I'd covered up my cowardice with ingratiating platitudes. Reddening, I sensed the only judgement here was disappointment when someone fails to do themselves a favour.

Suicide was never far from the room. It loomed over it just as the Humber Bridge hangs over the city, and the two are very much entwined. For a place as deprived as Hull the Bridge stands like a terrible temptation. One guy in the group said he had made a break for it at the weekend, only to save himself by blurting out his intentions to a group of lads drinking nearby. I shrank further into my shell. Suicide scenarios had played on the screen behind my eyes non-stop for years. I was all right these days, of course. Apart from the breakdowns, heavy drinking and all-consuming fear of other people. Having begun dismantling masculinity at *The Book of Man* I'd mostly succeeded in dismantling myself.

Even that was a half-truth. I was here for a reason. To reveal the thing I always keep hidden.

It was my turn again, this time to answer the upbeat final question: 'Where have you always wanted to travel to?' I began stuttering, on the verge of ignoring the question and blurting out *the thing*. Another one of those alarmingly fast tides of emotion rose up, with honesty surfing on the crest. Years of man-lifeguarding came to my aid: I said something about Centre Parcs and passed the ball on.

The facilitator declared the meeting at an end and caught me with a sympathetic eye as he talked about extra meet-ups for a game of football. Clearly I wasn't hiding my discomfort as well as I thought. Despite barely revealing anything, I had exposed myself far too much. As soon as the door opened, I was out of it, chasing myself away.

In the car I took a route avoiding a view of the Bridge.

In 2019, 94 men a week killed themselves in the UK. How many more men out there aren't talking but need to?

In a survey by the men's health charity Movember, 30 per cent of men in the UK said they didn't feel comfortable talking to their mates about their mental health problems, but 60 per cent said they'd like to help their mates with theirs. If anything sums up the absurd predicament facing men today it's this. Everyone wants to be the shoulder to cry on, but no-one wants to cry. Men sense they need to change but, because no-one wants to go first, we carry on in a merry conspiracy of mutual misery.

Depression was something I'd only ever sought help for half-heartedly – a sleeping-pill prescription handed out by an aloof GP, a series of counselling sessions at university. Instead I reconciled my problem by diagnosing myself publicly with a condition called 'miserable Northern twat'. This provided a means for people to fathom the awful silence into which I so frequently sank. Truthfully, I couldn't understand why tear-sodden breakdowns were regular occurrences, why my daily life was undertaken with a black fog inside my head, why I was too afraid to talk to anyone. When it came to my mind, I had no concept of anything diagnosable. All its tortuous twisting was simply the way I was. A weirdo. I kept up a certain grinning front at work and avoided drawing any attention to myself. Lamentably, other men in my orbit were almost certainly doing much the same.

What has become known as the Mental Health Crisis does not only affect men, but for them it represents an important breakthrough in providing the end of a thread by which you can unravel masculinity. This is because mental ill health in all its forms – whether it's depression, anxiety or eating disorders – is at odds with everything society tells us a man should be. The male ideal is about strength, stoicism, being in control. It is not only uncomfortable for men to express feelings other than rage; it is also transgressive. Shocking to witness. If a woman breaks down in an office, other women will rush to support her. If a man collapses in tears in the office the other men will back the hell away, repulsed, trying not to catch it.

It follows that unravelling masculinity is crucial if you want to deal with mental health effectively, which means stripping away the usual personas to allow vulnerability, beyond which is revelation. Mental health engagement allows you to think through what made you the man you are. In turn, serious self-analysis provides a profound approach to mental health problems that are often the result of a tangle of issues unable to be solved by throwing pills at the problem.

On the way out of Hull I drove past a bomb site from the Blitz when the Luftwaffe devastated this crucial port city. Curious how a number of these sites have been left like scars, so old wounds are never forgotten. To have men's mental health on the agenda in this hardened area is a powerful change.

Men's tendency to suppress emotion may be viewed as an admirable trait – not simply in war, but when pushing on through life's daily pressures. Yet, as with many aspects of masculinity, the positives can lead to negatives. Serious life trauma can often go unacknowledged and unreconciled. Even if the problems gnawing at your insides appear manageable – perceived inadequacies compared to others, hatred for the body you were born in, or a career path that feels desultory – when you swallow your disquiet it can curdle into misery.

Often the suppression is taken at face value, though – is just considered to be The Way Men Are. Cold bastards. After the First

World War psychiatrists were surprised to discover the mental traumas of soldiers they had considered to be intractable warrior types. The severe mental symptoms of young men emerging from the horrors of the battlefield ended up grouped under the term 'shell shock'. Such assumptions are hard to shake even today, which is understandable: only a couple of generations back being a man really did involve putting on your boots to go and kill Nazis. Not only do such assumptions persist, however, but they are also idealized, as the standard male modus operandi to be drummed in from nursery age.

Today certain voices in society still insist that, without a war to define us, men have become lost. In our tumultuous digital age, where new technologies are destabilizing work, social and moral structures, both wars maintain a grip on the popular imagination because of their perceived solidity. In England you can't go five minutes without hearing the slogans 'Our Finest Hour', 'the Dunkirk Spirit' and 'Keep Calm And Carry On'. War is oddly comforting here: not the horror, but the pride, the defiance, the victory, the clarity of right and wrong. For men, the war persona, the noble warrior, is still held in the highest regard. While the bravery of the old soldiers is rightly lauded, the warrior-hero ideal glosses over the real humanity of those men, whose emotions of fear, grief and panic were unquestionably just as much a part of the struggle.

After the First World War, Sigmund Freud's nephew Edward Bernays – usually called 'the father of public relations' or 'the father of spin' – took some of the psychoanalytic insights of his uncle, along with wartime propaganda techniques, and applied them to mass marketing; promoting smoking to women ('Torches of Freedom'!) was one of his big hits in the 1920s. As Adam Curtis's documentary

The Century of the Self reveals, Burnays was instrumental in revolutionising the way products were sold, by tapping into the unconscious desires of the genders, or simply telling them what their secret desires were. In the economic reconstruction that followed the Second World War, a booming consumer market was founded on fuelling a new dream of individual fulfilment. For men, this meant retaining the warrior ideals lingering from the war to depict them as heroic breadwinners fighting for money and power. Men belonged to the workplace, not the home, were professional not emotional. This created a shared dream of the qualities such a man should possess, along with suggestions for how he could acquire them. A masculinity established by the narrative of war was taken up by marketers and plastered on billboards; it has barely changed since. Consequently, men look back at what we once were, instead of forward to what we could be.

An indication of the suffocating pressure of twentieth-century male fictions is how many men have grabbed the chance to behave differently now talk about mental health is flourishing. Ten years ago Andy's Man Club wouldn't have existed. Things are changing. They must. Men have become seriously dysfunctional despite – in fact, because of – the conditioning as to what a man should be.

A week later I was back in London, feeling the same kind of alienation I had blamed Hull for, while blanking the obvious conclusion that it might not be these places that were the problem, but me. Instead I was stewing on London as an Imperialist relic, a dusty façade concealing a playground for self-interested hyenas feasting on the fears of its populace. Great people, I told myself, can achieve great things here, but only by fighting every second for a grain of truth within the crush of arseholery.

Extinction Rebellion had disrupted the transport system, so I walked from the City to East London through the invisible fug of masculinity: the streets thronged with men like me, head down but eyes to the side, observing their place. At Bank the suit was the marker of your assimilation, though now augmented with sleeve tattoos peeking out and extravagant facial hair; signs of an identity crisis, a conflicted self-awareness. By Old Street American workwear was the dominant aesthetic; I was dressed in the same manner, with turned-up jeans, heavy boots and plaid shirt: a bizarre middle-class English adoption of the stripped-back maleness of Texan oil rig workers. 'Accept me!', I desperately screamed – in a casually downbeat manner.

The fashion was trying a touch too hard, but it was the restless eyes that told the story. Look more closely at the men with coffees gripped in their hands, their gym kit stuffed in their laptop bags, the solo lunches on park benches, and you can detect simmering anxiety. Depression can floor you, but its main trick is to allow you to continue living, despite a vortex of panic destroying your insides. It may be at half-speed, but you can function.

Seeing the demoralized body language, it made me wonder what the psychic effects of the broad cultural debate around 'toxic masculinity' had been; a panic about male identity that men hadn't really dealt with yet. Possibly because of the scope of the problem, a suspicion that sexual harassment was just one creeping branch of a rotten tree of masculinity. The black fruits of which were violence and suicide. Which then only led to harder questions: was society in decline, its brutal systems and narrow expectations acting as the putrid soil feeding this tree?

Or was I simply projecting this, inventing an imaginary tree to piss onto while the majority of men were carrying on as usual?

13

Hard to say, but I was on the way to meet a man who could give me some insight into this through his personal and professional mental health experiences.

I'd arrived at my destination, snapped back into the real world with the sudden alarm of impending human interaction. The hotel bar was chintzy, authentically unauthentic. I took a blue velvet booth, with a large silver mirror tilted above it so you could look down on yourself. All clear. I hate mirrors, but I'll hate them more when there's a bald patch staring back at me.

Jonny Benjamin MBE was late, providing an opportunity for guilt-free screen time. I swiped through the #masculinity thread on Instagram:

Masculinity makes her wet/
Masculinity isn't toxic. It's men who aren't masculine who are toxic./
Get you a WOMAN, who wants to listen to you, learn from you, see you win, support your visions and fall in love with you daily./
If you think lifting weights is dangerous, try being weak. Weak is dangerous./
All it takes is a beautiful fake smile to hide an injured soul and they will never notice how broken you really are – Robin Williams/

In the UK, one in four people experience mental health issues every year. It's the second largest burden of disease, responsible for 72 million days lost, costing £34.9 billion. More women than men experience mental health problems, but three times as many men take their own lives. Data from the suicide-prevention charity CALM indicates that this is because men avoid reaching out for help, and their suicide attempts tend to be more violent, more final, than women's. Such insights suggest masculine expectations steer men to extremes in their mental health struggles.

Jonny arrived in a whirl of mortification, quickly gathering himself for another interview delving into his darkest moments. He had entered the public consciousness in 2008 after he was talked down from jumping off Waterloo Bridge by a passer-by, which resulted in a media campaign to find the identity of the Good Samaritan. The story, told in his book *The Stranger on the Bridge*, was a key moment in bringing male mental health to wider attention, along with the shortcomings in services to help those struggling.

'The education and health system are geared to be reactive to mental health,' said Jonny, 'rather than looking at prevention. The waiting lists are a scandal here, with the average time from diagnosis to treatment ten years. It's shameful, and even harder for boys and men. Men are more likely to die by suicide, but the drop-out rate for men in mental health services is huge. Even if they get to a doctor in the first place, the system is not set up for them.'

Jonny's personal experience within the care system was fraught with difficulty, not least scepticism.

I went to my GP for the first time when I was 17, and said I was suicidal, but it was months until I heard from the counselling service I was referred to, by which time I thought university would sort me out. I did go to my student GP a number of times there, but it was never taken seriously. The doctor said, 'You're a student, you're drinking too much, you're not eating well, you'll grow out of it . . .' Then, when I finally had a breakdown and was put in psychiatric hospital, everything was so clinical. They'd observe you, not talk to you. This is why I ran away to the bridge: I couldn't take it any more. And it's how this guy on the bridge saved me. He gave me this human connection. He wanted to talk. And listen.

The stranger on the bridge turned out to be a personal trainer called Neil Laybourn. One of things he said to Jonny as he dangled over the Thames was, 'I really believe you're going to get better, mate.' That tender reassurance was exactly what Jonny needed to hear. In such moments any suggestion that all men are toxic bastards is easily refuted. Indeed, part of the value of mental health campaigners talking about their experiences has been the way they've been able to celebrate men's 'softer' sides. Jonny and Neil's story helped mental health reach the top of the national agenda, soon aided by royalty, sports stars, actors, musicians and public figures of every kind sharing their own stories. Jonny has been in high demand as a spokesperson, but I was surprised to hear that, from his position in the eye of the storm, he sees a lot of talk but not a huge amount of structural change. 'We see lots of famous people in media talking about it, which is great,' he said, 'but we need actual support services. Companies are ticking boxes, with sessions on World Mental Health Day, but it should be present all the time. I get fully booked up on that day, but when I ask companies if I can come in two weeks later, it's a no.'

Jonny sees this as reflective of a society built on restrictive views of males which are very hard to shift. 'I was really sensitive as a small boy,' he said. 'Then, when I got to six or seven, that's when I got the message of "Jonny, you're getting a big boy. Big boys don't cry." It causes boys to suppress their emotions and vulnerabilities.'

Assumptions are flawed when it comes to boys. On the occasions when I've braved school trips with my young son's class, you can see more obvious disruption than with the girls. However, it's not mindless action at the expense of emotion; rather, it's because emotion is right there, on the surface: irrepressible enthusiasm, puppyish scrapping, giving way to hot tears of rage and regret. It is an unfiltered life, but it is far from animalistic; nonetheless, we train boys out of their expressiveness. Granted, teachers have to get through the day without murdering anyone, but we don't seem to know what to do to help boys mature their emotional responses. Instead, we shut the 'naughty boys' down.

That process begins at home, Performative 'hardness' from influential adults can mean 'wimpy' feelings are denied altogether unless it's in certain specific situations. 'When I was young,' Jonny recalled,

> I used to watch Crystal Palace with my dad. It was a nice bonding time, but I found it weird that during the match the guys around us would be really open – when they scored they'd hug and kiss you, and when they lost, they'd sometimes cry. But as soon as you're out the stadium, you shut down. From a young age you see there's only certain places you can show emotions.

Like Jonny, I was a 'sensitive' kid who quickly realized that sensitivity held no social currency for boys. When it manifested itself in others it was often punished by exclusion or physical pain. Sensitivity, emotions, had to be hidden. Because boys all come to this understanding you all think you're the only one experiencing them. Boys become expert at pretending they don't feel, in order to fulfil the coveted, and obtuse, ability to 'get on with it'. There is some evidence to suggest that baby boys are actually more emotional than girls (a study entitled 'The Fragile Male' found boys' brains in the womb were more reactive to maternal depression and stress), though it may simply be the case that males are like everyone else. It's not that men don't have emotions, don't feel the lows: it's that five minutes after birth it becomes socially unacceptable for them to show it.

Default Male clichés have produced this strange conception that men are this highly rational, very reasonable breed, and everyone who isn't a man, including non-hetero men, is weird, flighty and over-emotional. Yet look at, say, one of the most disastrously far-reaching events of our era, the financial crash of 2008. Blame was placed on Wall Street traders giving in to what economists call 'animal spirits', something conventional notions of capitalism can't account for. In other words, they acted irrationally, panicked and brought about ruin. You might say masculinity was responsible, or at least a distorted masculinity that insists on men always being in control, leading to bizarre pressures to never fail. The inevitable result: moments of catastrophic madness. It happens on Wall Street, in family homes, in governments and in pubs: everywhere today you can almost hear the tense vibration of an internal wire about to snap.

Jonny now mostly works in education. Mental health problems in young people are creating a demand which underfunded local authorities can't meet. 'Seventy-five per cent of young people aren't getting the help or support they need,' said Jonny. 'And they're the most vulnerable in society. So many of the people in prisons started as young offenders, and 95 per cent of prisoners are male. You just know that if they'd had the right amount of mental health support when they were younger, it'd be different.' Part of the difficulty Jonny faces in his work is that many parents seem frightened of exposing children to mental health matters, with the result that boys are left alone and put even more at risk.

Then there are religious complications. 'I'm from Jewish culture,' said Jonny. 'My family came from Europe to settle in the UK, and particularly with the men everything is suppressed, all the anti-Semitic violence and trauma. Since the world wars we know that men came back and stayed stoic, and that's passed down the generations, I'm sure.' Jonny leaned forward to cup his coffee:

> Sexuality can add another layer of shame if you're a gay man. For me it was linked to religion, and was another reason I ran away. I couldn't admit it – I saw it as a failure, like a sin. Straight guys find it hard to understand how easy it is for them; it is accepted. In the 1940s you could go to jail for being gay, and there's still culturally a resistance. Vilification of the trans community has become almost accepted – I find it very shocking.

A further difficulty is that children can be afraid of what's going on in their own heads too. For anyone, it is hard to admit you have issues, but for inexperienced minds with no perspective on how things might change, it can feel as though one is intrinsically damaged. Denying problems comes from terrified self-protection. With parents, teachers, employers, governments, universities also ignoring this tricky problem, there is a conspiracy of silence. Despite the resistance, Jonny has had tangible success finding things that work for little kids. 'We created the world's biggest mindfulness class, with primary schools around the world. Concentration, behaviour and general wellbeing improved after doing just that one class.'

Nonetheless, Jonny left me with his fears about a mental health backlash. He and many others in this field have found themselves on the receiving end of abuse by macho media commentators and sweaty trolls, deriding mental health talk as whining by the molly-coddled. 'The backlash has involved a doubling down on wanting to return to the idea of strong men again. Certain old-school figures criticize men who don't fit into their idea of what a man can be. I can only put it down to people feeling very uneasy about a new world of gender relations. We want to hear more from the good men, not these old guys sucking up all the attention.'

On my walk back into the centre of London I was mulling over whether the Mental Health Crisis marked a mass outbreak of mental health problems, or if people were suddenly talking about issues that have always been present. The backlash works on the latter assumption: that young folk today are simply too soft to handle life. While the most casual look at the past, at Van Gogh or *Hamlet*, will show mental health problems to be nothing new, our time exerts unique pressures only the most disingenuous sceptics would dismiss – most obviously the live human experiment of the smartphone era, recasting us as rats tapping at screens for algorithmic treats. Scientists have raised concerns about the impact of digital technology on the regulation of emotions, attention spans and anxiety: rapid-reward cycles, over-exposure to news, multi-tasking in which a screen is always present and a lack of face-to-face communication: all play a part. Yet there is no firm answer; studies are too inconclusive to brand the bombardment of our lives by technology and social media as 'bad'. At the very least these networks provide the opportunity to find like-minded people and, on the issue of mental health, a voice to counter the backlash.

I thought of Ben West, a mental health activist I'd met for coffee the week before I spoke to Jonny. His brother had died by suicide the year before at 15 years of age; Ben was 18. In the terrible aftermath, Ben found an outlet for his grief on social media, along with a purpose: to help prevent more deaths. He launched #WalkToTalk to encourage people to open up while exercising, and successfully campaigned for the UK to appoint the first Minister for Suicide Prevention. 'Teachers still aren't being trained in dealing with mental health issues,' he told me.

> Students who are depressed often become withdrawn, which makes them easier students. They can get forgotten. We're now working on a #SaveOurStudents campaign, fundraising for mental health training packages for schools and universities. The government hasn't listened to our petitions to date, so we'll wake them up with this campaign.

Like Jonny, Ben is tackling head-on the major indicator of a degrading society: rising mental health problems among young people. While here the authorities generally disregard such matters by focusing purely on digital issues – 'Cut down on screen time, guys' – in America the matter has been taken seriously by the scientific community, which has gone beyond linking the trend with social media exposure to link poor mental health to life after the 2008 crash and 'the Great Recession'. Generation Z have followed millennials into a world marked by rising inequality, declining economic mobility and increased poverty. One scientist from Stanford University called millennials the 'canaries in the coalmine' for toxic economic trends, reporting them as more likely than previous generations to die prematurely from suicide or drug overdoses. Between 2008 and 2016 mortality rates among 25- to 34-year-olds increased by 20 per cent, driven mainly by suicide and drugs. This trend is echoed in the UK, where millennials hit what should have been the prime of their career during the recession, to find themselves instead fighting for survival in a lost decade of longer working hours and stagnant wages. Dubbed 'Generation Rent', a third of millennials, figures suggest, will never own their own home. Add to such non-existent prospects the government's 'austerity measures' – deep public spending cuts to welfare, support services and housing, aiming to reduce budget deficits caused by bailing out the banks, which hit the poorest hardest (the use of food banks in the UK doubled between 2013 and 2017) – and there have been predictably serious consequences for mental health.

Between 1981 and 2007 there had been a downward turn in suicide rates in the UK, until an increase in 2008. While the figure has fluctuated since, in 2018 suicides rose again: males aged 20–24 saw a 31 per cent increase in suicides year on year, while suicides among females aged 10–24 hit the highest ever recorded. Those figures continued to increase in 2019. The highest number of suicides have remained among men in the 45–49 age bracket, but it is rising alarmingly among the young. In a time of so many 'social determinants' for mental health problems combining, it's obscene that the young are sometimes branded attention-seekers when it comes to mental health. Kids are killing themselves in greater numbers because older generations have screwed the world.

Mental health is not merely a personal issue. The fight for better mental health is both an individual one and a larger social struggle; the two are intrinsically knotted together.

A heavy door to a private members' club in Soho was in front of me. I was here to meet another leading light in mental health, who aims to contextualize inner struggles to help men escape their personal hells.

Poorna Bell had already secured a quiet area for us to talk, which she was rigorously policing by pushing yah-yahing clientele out the fire exit. A journalist, weightlifter and author, she wrote a book called *Chasing the Rainbow* about the suicide of her husband Rob. It's a tale of how men hide their traumas away in shame because of the perceived failure to be the kind of man society demands.

'I feel the work being done around masculinity, around destigmatising asking for help and not seeing things as a weakness, really needs to be doubled down on,' said Poorna. 'It's about celebrating your peers who are tackling their own mental health problems.' However, Poorna recognized that even when such discussions are more permissible among groups of men, it's not easy to suddenly acquire the skills to make them effective. 'You're asking men to speak in a language they haven't been taught,' she went on. 'Even if someone wants help, how can you expect them to articulate that? If you're a man who is emasculated around expressing your emotions, there's a missing link.'

She believes there needs to be a personal interrogation by men not to simply understand their pain, but create new modes of living beyond the comforts of Default Male territory.

> If you're not having a constant check of the things in your life and what things actually suit you as a person, that's scary. To base your worth on something your parents may have taught you is too rigid. I think that the sense of absoluteness in men is a problem. I feel like it might be helpful if there could be an injection of fluidity into masculinity. Which would mean, if you decide not to follow a particular path in life, you will still be accepted.

If we men are made into insecure creatures asked to deny parts of ourselves, then it follows that we are very much influenced by peer groups where affirmation is found and acceptable behaviour learned. You'll do anything to be included to avoid ridicule, so you find common ground on accepted interests to maintain the rigours of masculinity without having to reveal what's behind the mask. Walk into the roughest pub in the country and talk football, and you'll be all right. Walk into the poshest pub in the country and talk anxiety, and you'll be ridiculed. Men police one another on exhibiting old male standards, or connecting with societal stereotypes of masculinity, in an insidious way. To pass the tests, you project yourself as in control even when you're drowning. 'This idea that fallibility is the worst thing . . .' mused Poorna: 'that's not actually how human beings work. I feel we should operate from a place where, if you show fallibility, the consequences don't have to be completely linked to your sense of worth as a person.'

A couple of years ago I lost my job, and unexpectedly found myself a stay-at-home father and partner with no hope of further employment – mostly because I nursed my shame so carefully that the idea of applying for a job was unthinkable. This downward spiral was compounded by my pariah status. Men's mates, well-meaning as they might be, stay at a remove: the old repulsion. We are so invested in keeping up a pretence of emotional control that it's disturbing to witness other men losing their grip: *There but for the grace of God go I.* With my own situation it was mutual avoidance anyway: I chose to isolate myself in order to feel the weight of failure. I deserved it, I felt, and pursued it further. Smart.

Poorna doesn't particularly believe there are inherent self-destructive traits in men: more a disturbing gap in male communication which shuts down just when they need it most.

'I just think we're the product of the environments we are raised in,' she said.

> With my generation and the ones above I see a blank in the men, an inability to communicate how you're feeling. That leads to self-destruction: self-medication and violent behaviours. When you look at the gender disparity of the prison population that is incredible. I believe every single person has the capacity to be good and bad, but I think that's down to how you're shaped and what you're exposed to.

Am I good or bad? For the longest time, I thought I was an innocent in the world, pure of heart, trying his best to be a nice person: a common trait in indulged men, I think. I could maintain the 'nice' self-image even as my depressive episodes saw my behaviour deteriorate, with self-medication and complete emotional withdrawal ruining relationships. None of it my fault. When the possibility arises that you might not be a good person, I found, it becomes not a moment of redemption but a cue to dive into the lake of fire you've created. Self-hatred triggers a sudden urge to put partners, jobs, health, everything, at risk because you feel you don't deserve any of them; you become a finger poised over a big red button. Poorna linked this to the key issue of male shame: 'By shame I mean being constantly fearful about how you are perceived as a man. A lot of the arrogance comes out of this undiluted fear of people thinking that you're not worthy.'

I asked her how this had played upon her husband, Rob.

'Rob was pretty confident about who he was, but I didn't realize some of it was bravado covering really deep insecurities,' she said.

There was a lot about him that I just didn't know, that he didn't want to show me because he was ashamed. A consistent feature of his life was he wouldn't say when things were going wrong. It was shame. He felt he wasn't ticking the boxes about being a man that he was supposed to. For instance, he signed up to a gym membership and only went twice. I thought he was being lazy, but when I got to the bottom of it, I realized he felt intimidated in the weights section. He was 6 foot 2 and broad, Martin! It would never have occurred to me.

Rob developed a secret drug habit which exacerbated his mental distress. I asked Poorna what stopped him reaching out.

'Rob actually had a very insightful view of his behaviour,' she said,

but the paradox is it was also met with this unbelievable wall of denial that was insulating him against the reality of the situation: he was putting us through hell. The problem with the denial mode, where things weren't so bad even though everything around him was in flames, was it became a massive blocker to him actually getting help. There was a level of disengagement because he felt he could fix it. What I wish for him is that something had broken through the wall of denial. Just in the click of your fingers he'd be in a mode of: 'Everything is fine . . .'

I left Poorna thinking of the heavy role of gender in the knot of mental health causes. Weren't the extreme mental health symptoms in men the inevitable byproduct of a society training them not to feel? What a bitter irony that the standard, 'default', human being is supposed to lack humanity.

Deep in his heart every man longs for a battle to fight, a beauty to rescue, and an adventure to love/

26

Not all men are trash but most men I've met are trash/
Masculinity isn't toxic, a godless society is./

I was in invisibility mode on the train up to Sheffield, just another cishet fuckboy covered in muffin crumbs. I thumbed to a YouTube video from *The Book of Man's Mental Health Workshop* event. There I was on stage, half-turned from the audience, holding a mic in such a way that it kept me in shadow. Not a born performer.

Beside me, Professor Green was trapped in a projected illustration of his own face. He took over to talk about the difficulty of maintaining the public image of a tough-talking rap star when you have hidden personal problems to deal with. Everything changed for him when he made the BBC documentary *Suicide and Me* about the death of his father. In it, he talked to his nan about the suicide for the first time, and broke down in tears when he was shown an unseen photo of himself that captured the pure joy of a young boy in the arms of his dad. It was a heartbreaking moment. 'I've never actually watched *Suicide and Me*,' he revealed,

> but my friend Felix, who I've known since I was about six, watched it. He called me, upset, but he said, 'I feel like I know you so much better now. You make so much more sense.' Because we had never had those conversations, he'd never seen sides of me that he saw in that documentary. That was the beginning of it all for me.

Pro, real name Stephen Manderson, become a patron of the suicide prevention charity CALM as he forged a new path for himself as a respected voice on mental health. He said he'd noticed huge changes in how this has been perceived.

Up until recently there was no conversation. Everyone was still putting plasters on things. No-one was very vocal about struggling, because I think a lot of people weren't even aware of having problems, myself included. Now I go into schools, prisons – places where you wouldn't expect a conversation around mental health to be going on. When I was a kid the term mental health didn't seem to exist: you were just 'mental'.

Like Jonny Benjamin, Pro was conscious of those in positions of power being keen to discuss mental health, but less active when it came to making actual change.

I was at [accounting firm] KPMG for a talk and, because I'm lippy, I said to the bosses, 'It's all well and good having these discussions, but it's on you now to start acting on them.' Because if you want to make people aware that it is OK to be forthcoming about your mental health conditions at work, and there's no punishment or shame, then you need to have the support in place.

Part of the difficulty is generational, he thinks:

There are some people who come from an age where you pull yourself together and get on with it. A generation survived things like that – although my dad didn't: he took his own life because he couldn't pull himself together. But for a lot of people that's the only way, which is the negative aspect of the people that we have in senior positions in a lot of companies. So we need to inform, we need to encourage, and we need to make change.

I nudged the video to where Stephen recalled a phrase he'd grown fond of – 'Don't believe everything you think' – and talked about the temporal lobe of the brain which deals with fight or flight: how it can become over-stimulated when you're dealing with the chronic stress of today. He said, 'You start to deal with mundane situations with the heightened fight-and-flight part of your brain, meaning you're in a constant panic. With me it leads to catastrophizing. Creating disasters, worst case scenarios. So it's about relearning. Don't believe everything you think.'

I put my phone away. Absently picked at dried chewing gum under the table. Our impulses can't be trusted. It's a tough task to turn against psychological habits, though: to view our identities as potentially misleading constructions. Like finding out you're a replicant programmed to eat late-night cheese sandwiches and acquire flat-pack furniture.

The Mental Health Foundation says mental illnesses are divided into 'neurotic' and 'psychotic'. Neurotic symptoms are severe forms of 'normal' emotional experiences such as depression, anxiety or panic that anyone might experience at some time in their lives. Psychotic symptoms can interfere with perceptions of reality, affecting the way you think, feel and behave, and include bipolar disorder and schizophrenia. People suffering from psychotic symptoms will often suffer from neurotic symptoms too; there is no hard line between them.

Mental health problems are commonly misunderstood to be the result of chemical imbalance in the brain. Research by Harvard University recently refuted this, suggesting different forces interact to bring about a condition like depression, including faulty mood regulation, genetic vulnerability, stressful life events and medical problems. There are many millions of chemical reactions inside your brain's nerve cells (neurons) that are responsible for your moods and perceptions. Antidepressants work by boosting the concentration of neurotransmitters (the chemical messengers between neurons) like serotonin and dopamine. However, due to that incredible complexity of individual neurological activity, and because everyone has a unique combination of problems to deal with, medication can have a limited effect. Even 'psychotic' symptoms cannot be put down solely to brain function: there is no known exact cause of bipolar disorder, but evidence suggests environmental and social factors can trigger it as well as genetics.

As I would come to appreciate, poor mental health can often emerge as the product of an individual's environment, together with other intersecting factors. There's no escaping the fact that, while mental health problems can affect people from all walks of life, suicide rates are highest among men in the poorest parts of the country.

Only the recently beaten up don't love Sheffield. I took a cab to a colourful building where Brendan Stone, Deputy Vice President for Education at the University of Sheffield, one of the founders of mental health charity Sheffield Flourish and a board member of the Sheffield NHS Trust for mental health, was waiting. Friendly in a way that's alarming to anyone as rigid as me, Brendan took me to his office for sandwiches and a chat. At the time he was working with NHS England on the issue of restraint in mental institutions. 'I'm involved because of my own experience of being restrained in a mental hospital when I was 19, which profoundly traumatized me,' he said.

> I thought the five medical staff were trying to kill me – they filled me with anti-psychotics and tranquilisers so I couldn't swallow, one was sat on my chest so I couldn't breathe, and as I lost consciousness I thought I was dying. The reason they were restraining me was simply because I was in distress, crying uncontrollably. I became homeless after that. I was running away.

He told me it's quite common to find homeless people who have been brutalized in the criminal justice or mental health system: the destruction of their psychological safety can shatter entire lives. NHS England is trying to build up relationships within wards to understand what the catalysts for such an incident might be, 'without blaming anyone'.

Brendan works in the nuanced areas of institutional treatment where a greater awareness of mental health is confronting prejudices and old methods, to offer a better-equipped support system than Jonny Benjamin encountered. I found this reassuring; away from social media squabbling there are people like Brendan working professionally to understand the needs of sufferers. Naturally, following the issues to where they're most prevalent leads them to struggling communities in which masculinity can play a dark and heavy role. 'We had an event with Sheffield Flourish about young men, violence and mental health,' said Brendan. 'Talking about violence was also a way into talking about masculinity, I noticed. It was moving to hear working-class men or People of Colour from Pakistani or Somali backgrounds discussing violence and their own trauma, having witnessed someone be killed or injured.' Mental health problems were inevitable in such circumstances, but Brendan noticed an appealing shift in how the young men were regarding the 'pressures to be a certain type of man. I was very impressed by their kind of discussions,' he went on.

> I could never have had them when I was their age. Really reflective, thoughtful, aware. Sometimes being a bit macho, but also comfortable being vulnerable, saying they were scared or crying because one of their mates had been injured. They could be in both those spaces, and *that's* the sort of man I want to be.

Indeed. Sounds like the future. And really, it is about both talking and education: a concerted effort to study and support, starting, as Brendan said, with an appreciation of the diversity of mental health experiences. 'There are issues worth considering like levels of education, class, race, religion – all of those things will play a role in how a man responds to a mental health difficulty.'

This is not simply about encouraging individuals to cope with their mental health problems: it's about understanding community challenges and improving the environment to actually prevent them. It's not all in our heads: outward forces have an effect, politics has an effect, our country's whole way of doing things has an effect. Brendan put it like this:

> The material conditions we exist in determine the way we are as people. I'm not a socialist, and I don't put all the blame on Thatcher as some people do, but I think there are patently problems with free-market capitalism. It's important there is a regulation of the market, and intervention, to make sure our fellow citizens have a good standard of living – are able to build a life that is meaningful and productive.

It is a hard truth that not all mental health problems are created equal –something those of us from a relatively decent background should acknowledge, not to devalue our personal experience, but because some meaningful perspective will help us explore how to help others. 'If you go into one of the wards in Sheffield to talk to some of the men who are disabled by mental illness,' said Brendan,

> and then talk to some chap with a great life and plenty of money but who feels down . . . They may both have mental health problems, but these are worlds apart. Of course, the wealthy chap could perhaps get there – although to be honest the social determinants

of mental ill health mean he probably never would. He might have mental health problems, but he'd have access to resources that would enable him to manage it in a way that the guy on the ward from a working-class background wouldn't be able to.

Decreasing mental health problems in society is not a question of scented candles or hot yoga. According to Brendan, what does make a difference is material circumstances, education *and* relationships with people; that was the key for him to get back on his feet after being on the streets. Still, Brendan tells me he wouldn't say he's recovered, and one change in how mental health treatment is perceived should be to see it as about management, not cure.

> The people who say, 'I was at the bottom, reached out for help, got therapy and now everything is OK,' are a problem. In my experience mental health isn't like that, and life isn't like that. Depression is like damaging your Achilles heel: you're always going to be vulnerable to it. It's about learning not to be afraid of it.

A week later I'd left home at 10pm to hit the streets of London. The starting line for the walk was up ahead, at the Royal Naval College in Greenwich, another bone-white mausoleum for the Empire. I shook off the gloomy mood. Tonight was not the night. People were gathering in defiance of the march of time, ready to steal an hour from under the nose of the Royal Observatory. The Lost Hours Walk had been organised by the charity CALM for the night the clocks go back – the lost hour being reclaimed by a thousand walkers to remember people lost to suicide.

I was thinking about Poorna's Rob. About Ben's brother, Stephen's dad, Jonny sat on the railing of Waterloo Bridge. Also about the mums, brothers, sisters, sons who had sent stories to *The Book of Man*, trying to make sense of their tragedies.

CALM is the reason why the statistic of suicide being the number-one killer of men under 45 in the UK has hit the public consciousness. Supported by the likes of Princes William and Harry, Pro Green, Romesh Ranganathan and Rio Ferdinand, the charity has stamped its mark on the mainstream. Famously, in 2018 it created 84 statues to stand on the roof of the ITV building: the number of male suicides in the UK every week, at the time. Simon Gunning, CALM's CEO, calls these suicide figures 'a litmus test of the wellbeing of society'. Like Samaritans it provides a helpline for people in distress, but its raison d'être is prevention of the root cause. This involves making sense of who we are: a humane approach that uses humour as a tool to acquaint people with such serious issues; CALM's full name is the Pythonesque, Campaign Against Living Miserably.

I spotted Simon near the start of the walk, grinning at the huge turnout. 'People imagine it's depressing working for CALM,' he reflected, 'but it is the best thing. It is funny, it is a laugh, as much as anything, because we want to combat suicide with *life*. Tonight, look at all this life! This is what we want.'

My colleague Mark Sandford, the co-founder of *The Book of Man*, was among this life somewhere. He'd Whatsapped me that afternoon.

- Have you done any training? It says on the app you need to do training.
- App?
- Yes.
- Training?
- Yes.
- No. And I'm eating McDonald's. You?
- No. And I'm drinking red wine.

Everyone did look well prepared: technical footwear, big coats, water bottles, that kind of thing. I'd dug out some trainers and put on my waterproof, but the only real concession I'd made to the cold was a hip flask full of cognac. Now I was scared. The walk was 20 miles, along the north and south banks of the Thames, from Greenwich to The Oval and back again. It didn't sound too bad, but now I was here seeing everyone limbering up I realised it could be a shock to the system. Especially for those of us who'd been on the red wine. As I gratefully received a CALM scarf and pinned a number to my top, Mark appeared out of the crowd. Even from 50 metres away I could see he was leathered. He smiled at me and it was like watching the lift doors open in *The Shining*.

How much have you had?

'A few bottles.' His piratical face glittered. 'But I'm fine. This should be fine.'

I agreed that it should be fine. It was 20 miles, but we were walking, not running. And we were men! We didn't need training. *Let's just crack on and win this thing!*

When the man on crutches passed us, it was time to admit we'd fucked up.

Every muscle in my body was spasming in agony, from eyelid to toe. Beside me, Mark was walking as though his legs had been put on backwards. We were every man who has cracked on in proud ignorance, hoping to fluke it. We were the volley from the edge of the box which goes out for a throw-in. We were the leap over a fence which snags a scrotum. We were the punch thrown at a wasp on the nose.

By this point we were four hours in, about halfway there. It was around 2 a.m. The length and nature of the route meant the Lost

Walkers could swell to a group of 15 or 20, but then thin out to four or five, and sometimes it was only us two. It meant that often we were not recognized as charity walk folk, only as dickheads in scarves. Earlier, one guy tried to shoulder into me as he staggered out of a bar, intent on a fight, until I deftly side-stepped him; you don't want to make the papers for the 'charity walk brawl'. Besides, I'm a wuss. Now another Untucked-Shirt Guy greeted us by the Houses of Parliament with 'Look at you fucking *cunts*.' Nothing like having cheerleaders.

What was this? More acting-out of Being A Man? It incensed me. All this thick-headed violence made me want to hit someone. Maybe it was time for me to finally rise up to bring vengeance to this filthy cesspit.

'Haribo?' Mark had the sweeties.

That's better.

I tried out some self-awareness, acknowledging that I was no paragon of virtue. I too have rage in me: vicious instincts to judge and condemn, at the very least. If you talked to those men who had hassled us once they'd sobered up what would you learn? Chances are, mental health problems, addiction, life disasters. Happy people don't act that way, do they?

Time spent talking to other people on the walk was the true heart of the night. Everyone had been touched by suicide in some way. On Waterloo Bridge Mark chatted to a man walking alone to remember his son. He was enjoying quiet time with him, the boy still very much present in his mind's eye. Out by the new-build residences of Surrey Quays a woman told us about the suicide of her brother, while her friend described working at the harsh end of mental health care in institutions. These things were shared with deep affection, and a spirit of determination to not let these lost lives disappear. Tonight these walkers were grateful for the chance to *do something* about what had happened, to spread the word on suicide prevention. Reclaiming the Lost Hour to remember loved ones was also clearly a way for people to release themselves from being frozen in time by the loss. It was an act of living for those left behind.

I still had some cognac left, but I didn't want it. Mark was back to his usual empathetic self. Being a mess wasn't funny anymore.

94 men a week don't make it.

In the course of my work I've heard a lot of people say they decided not to die by suicide because they didn't want to upset the people around them. That had always been a barrier for me. Never the thought: 'I deserve to live.' It has not been considered manly to care about yourself. The ideals of incredible strength and noble suffering without complaint can lead men to avoid doctors, shrug off any help at work, deny problems to friends. What I see much of, in myself too, is how you can become a joke to yourself, an ironic impersonation of a man, where disaster is coveted as a pre-emptive strike on anticipated failure. This is sometimes funny, then not funny at all, because it's based on a lack of self-worth. What do you really matter anyway?

Mental health problems are a sign something is wrong. They are not to be dismissed. Untangling them, instead of laughing them off, can be the key to transforming your life. Transforming the lives of others too.

A gang of scavenging foxes wandered past, unafraid, perhaps sensing one of us was about to drop. The bright lights in Greenwich were getting closer, the Naval College ready to welcome back its least brawny adventurers. The lights blurred, coalesced into what was either the finish line or the gates of Heaven. I smelled death, or was it hot dogs? Grinning with a saliva-less mouth, all skull, I managed to stagger over the line in a delirium of simultaneous success and failure. A medal was placed around my neck – lucky, as it was the only place left with any feeling.

As we drank our celebratory teas and contemplated cabs I worried about Mark. Not just his legs, but the deleterious effects of our relentless business, and the health of our relationship, too, which is similar to that of ET and Elliott: me the freak in the closet turning white, him the puppy-eyed public face telling everyone things are fine. One day I'll tell him I love and respect him.

When I told the driver in the Uber home what I'd been doing he handed me two bottles of water. He turned the heating up. Put on classical music. We didn't talk again, but his gestures said a lot. If men are locked up together in a prison of masculinity, they are at least tapping on the pipes with escape plans.

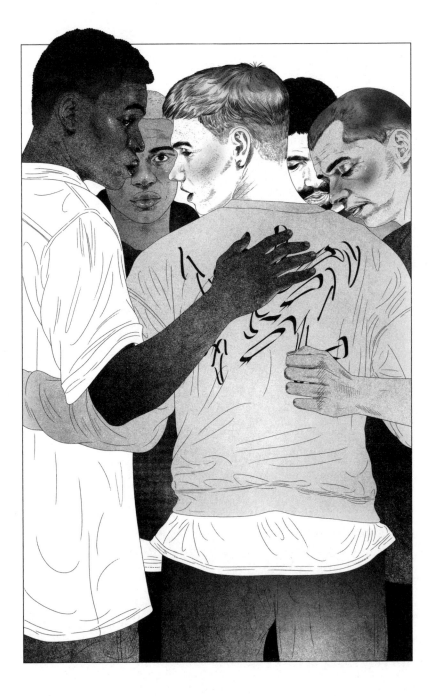

2

You Are One of the Lads

Tribalism and Masculinity

El Hombre Invisible. Blink and you'll miss him. Stare and you'll miss him. Just another white man making up the perpetual wall of the many.

Hanging off a rail in the Tube carriage I was no longer the person I was at home. Now I was a man in the world with all the others. They were inescapable tonight, a big Friday night: gangs of lads heading out in clusters of boiling intent, chanting, jeering, vaping. A few different 'types' were caught up in it – an old man on his own, two black women huddled together, another woman by herself staring at the floor. My instinct when it's this laddy and there's trouble in the air is to keep my head down and adopt the protective demeanour of apathy. If those men attacked the woman right now would I even do anything? I would. Surely I would?

The way white men can be invisible is different from how black men can be invisible, or the homeless, or women: their invisibility is about denial of rights, status, respect – their humanity. For white men, invisibility is about blending in with the massed ranks of those like you – those who have everything – to avoid losing that very ability to have everything. Masculinity is the lubricant of your conformity. You smooth off your edges, dress to fit the type, adjust your opinions to your peers, abide by the career path you fell into, keep the machine going without too much friction. No matter if you feel like you're losing yourself, selling yourself short in some way, or uncomfortable at witnessing some gross act of exploitation: you keep in line in the belief that one day you will reap the rewards. Any problems are to be dealt with in private, and understood to be strictly your own fault, your personal failure. What do you have to complain about anyway? Blend in. Be a Default Male. Be a good little bystander to your own life.

Stepping inconspicuously off the train at North Greenwich, at once losing myself in the crowd and cutting through it, I was desperate to escape. Up the escalators the chanting swelled to bursting point, but I was quickly out of the doors, following the guiding arrows on the curving wall into the cold embrace of the O2 Arena. The O2 celebrates itself as a source of national pride, even if no-one else does. By contrast, the hordes of men entering the venue now seemed less like the conformist droogs they did on the Tube and more like people lending a bit of chaotic humanity to a place seemingly designed to neuter.

I joined my friends in the Slug and Lettuce. Everyone was trying to get into the mood for the gig, which in this venue required nothing less than toxic shock. I stayed invisible, which didn't help with getting served. Later I joined the rest of the lads to chat about boxing, tunes, a bit about work – the usual. It can be hard to readjust to tribal dynamics but, when you're in it, there's enjoyment, warmth, familiarity. There's a lot to be said for it. Not a bolshy bunch, us lot, but maybe we looked like it if you were regarding us from across the room. Not everyone in the bar was white and male, but it was the majority. Many would see such a scene and identify it as the source of all the problems in the world – indeed, men themselves are now conscious of the vibe they give off. But what do you do? Ban male friendship?

When a director of the Chartered Management Institute declared in a radio interview that football chat should be banned from offices because it excluded women, it was hard to pick the most offensive aspect of what she was implying. That women don't like football? That conversations at work should be monitored? Or that anything with even a whiff of manliness is suspect? Somehow, though, it felt in tune with the times: just a rather extreme expression of the reassessment of what is acceptable when it comes to gender. Sexual harassment cases were seen as part of a broader culture of male dominance and behavioural entitlement. In the process has come – understandably, given the weight of history behind that culture – a demonization of men. 'All men are trash' has been the buzzphrase on social media, and some feminists are so sick of living in a man's world that they now call themselves womxn. Particular scorn is reserved for all-male groups, for they appear to present the biggest barrier to equality at work and respect in daily life, with the idea of the group itself serving only to embolden those in it and exclude everyone else. There's a latent threat in any all-male group, which is about territory, about dares, about wolf eyes and judgement. When you're a man in that group you feel the power of that threat: the buzz of those dares, the bond won by eviscerating what's outside. No wonder those who are on the outside find groups of lads obnoxious and threatening. All of this is blatant. But is there more to this than meets the eye – or indeed less?

In 2010 flint tools were found in Happisburgh in Norfolk that were dated to around 900,000 years ago. They would have been used by early humans called hominoids, who are likely to have utilized fire and worn animal hides. Yet Britain, then still physically part of the European continent, was only ever a stopping-off point for hominoids and *Homo heidelbergensis* and Neanderthals for many thousands of years. At the end of the Ice Age, in the Mesolithic era, rising tides simultaneously cut off Britain from the mainland and improved the climate enough to allow continuous human population by nomadic hunter-gatherers. While they would move around seasonally to exploit plant or animal resources, there is evidence of group settlements. Scientists studying such tribes now believe hunter-gatherer duties were shared by males and females, suggesting that there was an evolutionary advantage for groups with sexual equality: wider social networks, closer co-operation with other groups and a wider choice of mates. Flexible, mixed, tribes win.

This early population of Britain has been physically profiled using evidence from the uncovered skeleton of the Cheddar Man in Gough's Cave in Cheddar Gorge, Somerset. A Mesolithic hunter-gatherer who lived around 10,000 years ago, he had dark skin, long dark hair and blue eyes. If you're looking for the original Brit, that's him: Black – and beautiful. From about 4000 BC farming was introduced to Britain by immigrants from Europe, who still travelled around to forage for wild food, but during the Neolithic period erected monuments like Stonehenge, circa 2500 BC, around which a community could gradually gather. This trend was accelerated by a larger influx of Europeans, the Beaker people – named after the distinctive pottery that denotes the level of their development – whose DNA signifies that they had lighter skin, blue eyes and blond hair.

But they were latecomers. Black Britons were here first. Remember that next time any white Nazi 'nationalists' start bleating about England for the English. The English, sirs, were a mongrel race of immigrants from the start, from Viking hordes to Roman conquerors, to the Dutch, the French, Germans, Jamaicans, Persians – absolutely all of them rocked up on these shores to clash and co-operate, and swap fashion tips. Multifarious tribes grinding against one another to elevate the nation higher: that's the history of Britain. Or it was until the Empire and the international slave trade, when Great White fictions were scrawled over the past. The idea of white supremacy has always been a lie. Humans work most effectively through diversity. Successful tribes are never homogenous: they are in flux.

Successful tribes, not all tribes. Down at the O2 that night, dominated by Beaker drinkers, it was about formalized behavioural cues; not flux but solidity. Real things, for Real Men.

Pints sunk, fags smoked, coke snorted from credit card edges, bear hugs, scuffles, singing, chanting. 'Oasis! Oasis! . . . Oh, *sorry* . . . Liam, Liam, Liam!'

Concrete corridors clogged with sweating men. There had been a terror attack on London Bridge that day, so extra security procedures were delaying entry. In the queue most of us seemed to be trying to overcome middle age for the Liam Gallagher gig, at least for one night. Bucket hats bobbed, parkas flapped, lairiness was lauded and Mancunian accents were adopted. Trouble stirred as boredom struck. Chanting West Ham fans squared up to a couple of Spurs fans. A group with eyes like cue balls were getting in confrontations with inanimate objects: crowd barriers, a bin. When one fella failed to stare out a wall, he punched it.

Obnoxious behaviour, yes, but it all felt like a performance to me; not simply an exhumation of the 1990s but a chance to play with the rituals of traditional masculinity. Ones which I was by no means above – indeed, was enjoying: the drinking, the piss-taking, the crass jokes, the being a bit of a pillock. Part of it was 'blowing off steam', but not solely: while the rituals followed obvious 'hard' stereotypes, they were also gestures of belonging, of assent to the group, of reassurance. The performance was for each other's benefit, to show we were operating as we should within a male group, in a place like this, at an event of this nature: a lout-fest.

Yes, undeniably we were engaged in a gleefully ugly kind of schtick, which has often seemed to me – at gigs and in pubs, clubs, stadiums – to be an impersonation of working-class masculinity. No doubt there were plenty of genuine working-class folk present, but in such male-dominated environments there's a kind of unifying, swaggering, rebellious attitude that *plays* at lowness. This is an absurd but important factor in male behaviour: a tendency for men to aim to be 'lesser' than they actually are. Especially in England, because of the importance of class. There is a requirement to not get above your station, but also a romanticism about actually bending below your station which spellbinds plenty of nice middle-class boys and upper-class elites; as skewered by fellow 1990s alumnus Jarvis Cocker in Pulp's 'Common People'.

In England, being seen as ordinary is important, and for the men it borders on an obsession, one policed by peer groups. To not get too carried away with yourself. To not be pretentious. To play it dumb. The phenomenon of boys hiding their brains at school is well documented. Down it comes from fathers, and back up it goes into successive generations of men: an idealisation of macho boorishness. It operates at a level of politics – witness politicians sipping pints on the election trail, or indeed the entire boozy, nicotine-stained, belching persona of Nigel Farage, a self-styled 'man of the people' despite his background as a private school-educated stockbroker – where it belies a contemptuous insincerity because it plays upon class prejudice.

Such populism reeks of opportunistic image propaganda, rather than actually looking after the best interests of the people it claims to speak for. It frequently works, though. The 'real' pose pervades the collective consciousness. No doubt part of the appeal of Liam Gallagher is that he is 'real': even if he now lives in Hampstead, he's still seen as a working-class kid from an ordinary background who made it big in an unapologetic way. His untamed, unselfconscious masculinity always seemed like the dream: *He doesn't care what other people think.* He embodies a working-class purity in that sense, and is idolized by men of a certain age in a way that, say, Thom Yorke, isn't, for Thom Yorke comes across as uncomfortable, always trying to be something *different*. Liam *is* Liam. Or he plays himself very well, at least. It looks fun, and free. When so much of our identities feel compromised, men want a taste of what he has.

And here we were again, ecstatic with a ticket to be free for the night, intent on obliteration of the awkward self, a group of different people all doing 'real' as best we could. Which isn't to dismiss it: the rewards were genuine; within the agreed mutual act were expressions of friendship. Getting the old gang together for a shared experience. Like being stuck in a queue outside the venue when the gig you've paid for has already started. Vibrations were coming through the walls. He was on! But it was all right: we were together, and we locked into a bubble to forget about our troubles for a while.

Brotherly love is a romantic ideal hidden beneath the notions of the warrior ideal. You don't have to fight your battles alone, and you have someone to hang with during down time too. Don't let the heteronormative colly-wobbles deceive things: we call it brotherly love, but it's just love.

Love with limits, though. Where is the band of brothers when it comes to mental health? You'd expect buddies to help you out of a car crash, but what about helping them out of depression? There's not the urgency that comes with a burning wreck, but you can still lose your life to it. If we are seeing male suicide rising and mental health declining then you have to look at peer support: if we are so reliant on our tribes for happiness and self-image, are they failing? Are we too distracted by living up to the image of Real Men?

Studies have linked happiness and a longer life to maintaining friendship groups. Accordingly, men's inability to maintain friendships as their lives go on is seen as a major factor in suicides, and one of the reasons for men's lower life expectancy. Does the blind spot over mental health – easy to assuage with the solitary consolations of addiction – denote the fundamental limitation of male friendships? Because they don't go very deep, they are easy to lose. Certainly for the mental health charities reaching out to friends is a key part of their messaging. Men have received the message and want to help each other, but no-one wants to admit anything's wrong. Awareness has built; barriers remain. Who's the man to break rank, to establish a new behaviour to enrich the tribe?

By the wall, feeling the thud of the bass, I had to admit I'd been struggling for a while. Why couldn't I tell my friends? Knocked by the vicissitudes of depression, I had disappeared. Now I was back, after months away, but for how long? Not telling them what was really happening to me required a deception that only made me feel worse – but boring someone with my problems still felt indulgent. I mean, this is all supposed to be a laugh, isn't it? Affectionate, warm, fraternal, but not burdened by the heavy stuff. While this friendship of brave faces appears another link to the stiff-upper-lip war era, if you speak to military people – especially those who've been in conflicts – you'll find people who have shared deep emotional connections.

But all too often keeping in with male friendship groups means presenting a smoothed-over version of yourself, to the extent that your friends don't know you, and you don't know them, not really.

To get more of a purchase on the masculinity of male tribes today you can look at how the culture of work has developed over the past couple of centuries. Broadly speaking, before the Industrial Revolution there was a major artisanal culture, with men operating a trade close to home and raising their children to follow in their footsteps. With the call to the factory, however, came a split between home and work, and soon the delineation of work and the pub as 'male spaces', and the home and shops as 'female spaces', was set in stone.

There was a further separation to come: a rising middle class from which a certain type of professional man emerged. He rose out of local firms into bigger multinational corporations, a creature of the office adept at professional decorum to ensure he was an efficient member of a workforce. Technological advances only led to the loss of manufacturing jobs and more men entering, or supplying, offices. They didn't free anyone up – in fact, the hours became longer, and an understanding developed that even your leisure time was work time, and the pint after work with your boss and colleagues crucial to advancement. Your tribe became your work mates. Change jobs, change tribes. Travel light. No baggage.

Masculinity eased the tribal bonding with the idealisation of the old 'Alpha' type, this time in the guise of Corporate Guy. The Default Male with a 'proper job'. The kind of person who could rule meetings, keep a cool head while others flapped, and never splash Bolognese sauce on his suit. With a familiar combination of formal, manly gestures anyone could participate in the display of power, but ideally you'd be a certain type of well-schooled white man. Demonstrative trad masculinity was king; the actual work, as anyone baffled by the promotion of the laziest dickcheese in the building will testify, secondary.

In such environments, 'man up' meant: shut up and slog. Fallibilities were barriers to productivity, barriers to true shining masculinity. Generic male behaviour was encouraged in the observed settings of offices because it was easy to predict, reward and motivate. Women could join in too, in theory, if they embraced the same ethos. You had to blend in to the culture or lose your job. Be one of the boys or do one. *The Wolf of Wall Street* was a cautionary tale, theoretically. In actuality: pure working man's tribal fantasy.

Damien Ridge is a psychotherapist, social scientist and mental health expert. At his office at the University of Westminster I asked him to tell me about the key theories of masculinity that could shed light on male tribes. The first was 'hegemonic masculinity', a theory developed in the 1980s by the Australian sociologist R. W. Connell. 'It's the idea that masculinity is relational,' explained Damien: 'it's not within the man, it's between people. It's a whole social system.' Masculinity is, to appropriate the *Wolf of Wall Street* quote, 'fugazi … it's fairy dust, it doesn't exist': it only appears when people are rubbing up against one another. 'Competitiveness is built into the system,' he went on. 'You have the most honourable way of being a man, and all the subordinate ways of being a man underneath that then compete.' In recent times hegemonic masculinity has been taken to refer to the 'toxic' masculinity traits men become caught up in together, but Damien says it is often misunderstood, and the essence of the theory is the 'ideal' masculinity is most valued in any location, which could well have positive elements.

> Our research shows that men might be in a Buddhist meditation retreat where what's really valued is intimacy and compassion. But within that retreat there's going to be competition to see who can be the most spiritual. That's what Connell's saying: that there's always going to be an idea of winners and losers. Being better than other people is ingrained in the male psyche.

The theory challenged the popular notion of there being one natural, fixed masculinity. That was the lack I'd always felt, and what men's retreats seek and marketeers sell: an inherent manhood lost somewhere deep within; an inner Clint Eastwood that modern society has buried and we need to uncover, possibly through primitive rituals or by buying aftershave. Hegemonic masculinity said it's all relational: little point in acting like Clint Eastwood on the avant-garde jazz scene. (Mainly because Clint Eastwood is already there, but you take my point.)

According to the theory, the ideal values in any location can be subverted by the concept of 'resistance': where different models of valued masculinity could replace or alter those at the top through competing behaviours which challenge the status quo. Yet this exhausting scenario of continual fighting to prove or improve your position, in which weakness is intolerable and even relaxation unthinkable, has limitations, I think. Is it always competition, or does co-operation sometimes hold sway? Damien points out that many scholars now question the dominance of the theory of hegemonic masculinity. Certainly Andy's Man Club isn't a chance for dick-swinging, over who has the worst illness. Then there's self-sacrifice, as with the onlookers who banded together to battle the terrorist on London Bridge with a ceremonial sword and a narwhal tusk; you can't tell me they were competing for Hero of the Day. And what of wilful outliers – the loners who reject groups altogether; who purposefully seek exclusion in order to forge new values for living? Well what do those individuals ever achieve? Apart from Jesus.

Hegemonic masculinity is often cited to account for the perpetuation of a patriarchy which has established certain male values over a certain little domain: Planet Earth. If only us men didn't bristle at the term 'patriarchy', as though someone had just called *Rambo: First Blood, Part 2* an average film. 'Most men won't feel like they're in a patriarchal system,' Damien acknowledged,

> because they're at the very bottom of the heap. Think of the angry men (and women) that Trump appeals to, his base are disenfranchised. So men turn off from mainstream voices when they're not feeling the power they're supposed to have. We *must* live in a patriarchal system, because men are in control, but I don't think the majority of men feel they are getting anything out of it. If you think about it, it's a very small elite in control. If you use Connell's idea of hegemonic masculinity on a global scale (although Connell eventually admitted you couldn't really have a global hegemonic masculinity), you'll see most men are trampled by it. Even the ones at the top are damaged by patriarchy. The damage bleeds all the way through.

You can hear a women's orchestra playing the world's smallest violins striking up . . . But if the system is going to change, then men have to be shown that it only plays to certain characteristics to the detriment of all else; and for the ultimate benefit of the few.

One of the alternative ways of thinking about masculinity, Damien said, is to see it as performative. This approach comes from the American philosopher and gender theorist Judith Butler, who developed the idea that we repetitively *perform* gender to create the illusion that it is a solid thing, part of our identity. We act like the person we think we should be. As with hegemonic masculinity, there is no essential masculinity: rather it is something we act out, based upon information we pick up from the humans around us about the correct behaviour in that space. 'It's the idea that gender is not something you have,' said Damien: 'it's something that you *do*.'

Do men really leave the house, I wondered, deciding to act out being a man that day?

'I think you do, though,' retorted Damien.

> There can be a sudden transition. If you watch *RuPaul's Drag Race*, they have the ability to switch it on and become someone else, it is actually a new persona. It's the same for men going to work. The drag for an office might be a suit. You put it on, and then you put on a professional persona: you are not the person you are at home. These cues are really important. It *is* performative. It's about creating an illusion, but that is also a frightening prospect for some men!

The idea of performing gender is crucial when it comes to considering transgender people. Aside from the basic human right of being able to choose how to live your life, if we are all internalising and performing gender unconsciously from early on, then why complain if some people choose a different performance to the advertised show? Is the real reason why people are so offended that it reminds them that their own identity is so much crêpe paper and glue? The transgender community should be worshipped as the ultimate humans, for showing the rest of us how it's really done. If only it were so. The reality is our gender performances are brutally policed. If you don't perform in the 'real' way your gender should in a particular environment, there can be trouble.

'One of the first definitions of "doing gender" was by West and Zimmerman,' said Damien, 'and in their 1987 paper they said our competence as members of society is held hostage to our performances or how we do our gender. Think of "sissy boys" in the playground: the consequences for them can be brutal bullying.'

The performative aspect of masculinity has always been apparent to me. Trying to fit in, meeting ridicule, finding another route. In fact, our adaptability is nothing to be ashamed of. It's one of our true talents as humans, and supports the argument that masculine behaviour isn't standard for all men, everywhere. In Dubai, for instance, it is the norm for nationals to hold hands with their male friends when walking down the street. You wouldn't try that with your straight mate in Hull. However, kiss your gay male partner in public in Dubai, as you might back in Hull, and you can expect jail. Whatever your particular place has decided is 'normal' male behaviour is then vehemently defended as The Way Real Men Are.

Such thinking is deeply entrenched, because the instructions for behaviour in our environments are given every second we're alive, from parents, siblings, schools, films and ads. We suck it up to try to form an identity. For Damien the variations in gender behaviour around the world are proof that gender isn't biological, but to our psyches it certainly feels that way. 'I'm not saying it's not real,' he argued. 'The performance creates a reality for people from very early on – it's who we are . . . but there's a lot of fear and denial. Looking below the surface into the unconscious can be traumatic.'

Our friendship groups are critical in this respect: here the policing of gender performance is at its most acute, and bullying labels – 'sissy', 'pussy' and so on with variations continuing well into adulthood – can have lifelong consequences. In his psychotherapy work, Damien told me, he's seen that, while we are telling men to talk more, the actual experience of most men when they talk about their 'weaknesses' is that they face rejection: 'Research suggests men are very wary of opening up because of past rejection. They're looking for safety, non-judgement and not being pathologized.' To be a man who is accepted by the 'system' still too often means, therefore, being a man who will continue to reinforce the 'surface' of their personality without giving anyone a look beneath. For the 'good' of the group. Again, it's that sorry truth that men lose friends as they grow older, far more than women, because they have come through a culture of behaviour which prevents them from truly relating to each other. 'Most men in this country are on a trajectory to being more and more alone as they age,' said Damien. 'They're not trained to nurture relationships like women are. Men have to think about a new way of relating and being.'

Grayson Perry was in full transvestite splendour, towering in six-inch heels above the audience in the lecture hall. Before the domineering splendour of Grayson in full 'Claire' mode a Default Male can feel suddenly exposed as the drab enemy. The headline speaker at a conference at UCL called 'Engendering Men's Health', Grayson was delivering the thoughts on nostalgic masculinity he had first presented in *The Descent of Man*.

The strong warrior version of masculinity was needed in the pre-historical days, he said, but that's changed: 'It used to be utilitarian, but now it's decorative. It's ornamental, something to put on for a social occasion.' However, he rejected the notion of a current crisis in masculinity.

> It's always been in crisis, because it's always looking backwards. If you go back to the Industrial Revolution, people like William Morris worried machines would de-man the physical worker, so they grew beards and acted in this old-school manly fashion, because they thought masculinity was under threat. Whenever a fashion for beards crops up, it's when there's anxiety about masculinity.

Not that men were beyond hope. The key role models for men, he stressed, aren't famous faces, but the faces around us – 'because we learn most from the drip-drip-drip of everyday interaction.' When it came to any change, Perry positioned vulnerability at its heart:

> Basically, if you want to be happier, have good relationships. We are herd animals: we want company. In order to have good relationships you need intimacy, and to get intimacy you have to impact, and be impacted upon by, another person. This means saying stuff about yourself and asking the other person about them. Vulnerability is the key to happiness. I've found that if one man opens up in a group and says they've had a problem, the others all go, 'Oh, me too', and do actually talk. Often the barriers are in men's heads.

The next day I was on the phone to Robin Dunbar, Emeritus Professor of Evolutionary Psychology in the Experimental Psychology Department at Oxford University. Those studying the long game of human development do not have much patience with any idea that gender is socialized. Robin went so far as to call it 'complete rubbish'. The differences between men and women are biological, he said: 'There are sex differences, some more meaningful than others. Most are matters of degree: on average men are taller than women, but not all men are taller than all women.' But the most interesting, from his perspective, are social. 'The really big sex differences are in social behaviour,' he went on.

> They are really very consistent, very dramatic, and have very little to do with upbringing. You can tweak them a bit here and there, but boys will play in a very different way to girls from a very young age. That's true in monkeys and apes too. Monkey boys will preferentially select toys which we'd call stereotypically male. Monkey girls preferentially select toys we'd think of as girl toys. Dolls. There's no way that is a culturally induced effect. That's not to say that boys don't play with dolls, or that girls don't play with motorbikes, but on average there's clear-water separation.

He went on to say that

> Girls are much more social than boys. They have cognitively better social skills, as well as behaviourally better social skills. The major differences are in how they maintain their friendships. Girls do it by talking together; boys do stuff. What maintains boys' relationships is engaging in a physical activity together. With the best will in the world there's no way you are going to get boys to talk about their emotions together. Cultural things won't help. If one of them starts talking about his emotions they need to be laughed at by the rest. It is deep-rooted.

Robin has studied at length why male friendships aren't as long-lasting as female.

> They don't have a level of intimacy that girls' seem to. This is reflected in the way girls have an inner layer of these very intense relationships. If boys are in a romantic relationship that's the only

intimate relationship they have. If they aren't in a relationship they might hang out with a best friend. But, realistically, 'Jim' will be embedded within a group of four or five guys who meet regularly at the pub. It's very casual. If 'Jim' moves away, not a lot of effort is made to keep that friendship up. You just find somebody else to fill Jim's slot, and keep drinking. Anybody will do!

All of this was delivered by Robin with a chuckle, and the continual caveat that he was talking in general terms about averages for males and females. In individual experience there is always a 'spectrum' of behaviour where 'some boys are good at expressing their emotions and some girls aren't very good at it'. But he insists that you can only influence behaviour a little with interventions, and you can't 'make men into emotional, right-on people overnight'.

The vision of men as locked into the broad swing of our species was unnerving. I have a problem with genetic predestination, of limited options at the wheel of a biological speeding car, because it appears to limit personal responsibility. It also unnerved me because Robin's take on casual male friendships rang true for me in an embarrassing way. Indeed, while charities like CALM campaign for men to talk, they recognize that men are more likely to do so during shared, usually physical activities, and to create events where that can happen.

Does this mean, then, that we have to abandon ourselves to living out an evolutionary destiny of being a man? Not necessarily. A spectrum of masculinity means there is room for movement, and small changes can make huge differences as you're dragging men towards the emotionally connected end. That heavy weight of evolution can make the small problems of today seem unimportant, when they're not – they're all we have! Even if the most we can do is tweak, tweaking the suicide stats lower is reason enough not to be discouraged.

Which is not to devalue what Robin is saying. In fact, in dealing with masculinity it's crucial to view ourselves as part of humanity's stretch. Realistically, an interaction between primate impulse, chemical and hormonal idiosyncrasies, culture, memory, hunger, and plenty more, affect us at any one point. To dismiss any factor would be absurd, as would isolating only one – as I think often happens with evolutionary theory when it comes to men ('boys will be boys' etc.) – it all counts, the tangles matter, and any insight into the chaos can help with solutions to human problems.

Robin stressed that his research serves to inform how boys and men should best be educated: to understand them, not censure them. When dealing with the risk of suicide, he said, it's better to apply an evolutionary knowledge of men:

> This doesn't mean that boys' relationships, casual as they are, aren't important, because they seem to carry the same overall weight as the girls'. Therein lies the key with suicide: a guy who is destabilized by an event somehow needs to be kept in the loop with the other guys. This is not a crying-on-the-shoulder loop, which is what the girls would do: this is about pulling them out of the mire to go climbing mountains.

Proxy behaviour is more sophisticated than it seems, anyway. It may require a mountain to be climbed for men to talk, but what happens during the challenge? Is it possible that tenderness, co-operation, shared fears and vulnerability arise, not only in the actual talking but every treacherous step of the way?

Our lived experiences are made up of broad truths viewed from a distance, and smaller complex interactions. The tension between old values and new forms, between impulse and choice, acceptance and risk, is where all life's defining choices are made. It *is* life itself. No-one really knows how much we are shaped by genetic destiny and how much by lived experiences. What we do know is that we can attempt to get a grip on our own lives and let evolution take care of itself. After all, isn't the human struggle about the search for something higher than the natural states we were presented with? Leonardo da Vinci, Oscar Wilde, Stephen Hawking, Michael Jordan . . . what's real ambition about if not to transcend the limitations of merely being a man?

Once we were finally through the O2's security and inside the arena, everything was different, everything was all right. The sound destroyed the walls in your head and red lights strobed over laughing faces in the semi-darkness, bringing a delirium to the spectacle of bouncing bodies; in the altered moment either the music or the shadows unlocked a desire for intimacy. It certainly wasn't the booze, since there was only one bar, seven men deep; how could I get into the spirit of things without my liquid crutch? Then I was physically pulled out of my sulk into the masses.

While ostensibly everyone was there to see Liam, really we were there to be with each other. Men were doing a weird hug-wrestle-jump thing with each other, a bit of aggro-love, with much crooning badly into the nearest ear – it was tenderness disguised as laddishness, or laddishness flexing to allow tenderness. You couldn't be too cynical about it, a change had come over us, the self-conscious posturing lost to abandon.

Liam was singing the old hits, thank Christ, and the warmth between people was indicative of the comfort and sadness of nostalgia: the experience was a reminder of the puppyish days of free living before the adult male world got its claws into you. Great amusement could no doubt be found from witnessing grown men crying and singing 'Stand By Me' together, much as when grown men weep about a missed penalty – but, well, why not? At least emotion is proved to be there, and if most of the time men are performing a hardnut version of manhood you can understand the need finally to unleash that emotion, albeit in a pre-agreed blokey environment after fifteen pints of lager. Is it a dropping of the act? Not exactly, but it's the part of the act that's most joyful because it's least restrictive.

In such moments, or in their afterglow, you are able to talk about hope for the future, voice worries, find some reassurance. Chemically assisted or not, at least these kind of group activities still exist for men. If male friendship groups cause problems by suppressing expression, at key moments they can still flex. These groups may be dysfunctional, but, as Robin said, they must be maintained. I hadn't seen any of the people I was with for months. When was the last time I even went out? At a certain point I changed from drinking with friends, to drinking alone with friends present, to drinking alone. One day you look up and there's no one there at all.

Back in Sheffield, I was walking up one of those infernal hills in the student district. It was raining heavily, so I walked at speed until I slipped on some leaves. A couple of smokers outside the University Arms watched as I pulled myself together and resumed my journey at half the pace. That made me desperate for a repairing pint. Men don't fall over. Everyone knows that.

Dr Kitty Nichols was waiting for me in the lobby of the Elmfield Building. Kitty is a lecturer in sociological studies and an authority on men and masculinity: her PhD studied banter. As you'd imagine, she's one of the few to have taken it seriously.

'Men have emotions, but we don't read it that way,' said Kitty once we were in her office.

> We think men are emotionally inarticulate, but they're expressing it all the time. Banter is a way men are able to articulate resistance and emotion, and create dialogue and discussions, around subjects that they might not feel they're able to elsewhere. In a hyper-masculine sporting environment or workplace, men use the tool of banter because it's familiar in that space. And I argue men can use that tool to create change.

Kitty said she's interested in the nuances behind the clichés of male group behaviour; in how men in groups truly interact. When she was growing up her dad and brother were involved in rugby clubs, and when lad culture started to be heavily criticised she remembers being puzzled, because she'd seen things differently. Groups of man have a bad reputation for 'bantz', but it's not as simple as men just being horrible to each other: it can actually be about inclusion. 'At my rugby club', said Kitty,

> men often used banter to address something that was contentious. One of the participants had severe mental health problems of which everyone was aware. He told me that actually the way he felt able to talk about it was if someone took the mickey in some way. That was their way of saying, 'Are you OK to talk about this?' It opened up the space.

In male groups problematic behaviours readily occur, but they can be challenged: peer piss-taking is not simply to reinforce masculinity; when someone steps out of line it can also be a corrective. Kitty talked about witnessing a player in the rugby team make homophobic comments about another player who had turned up with his hair in a top knot: the rest of the players stood up for him to bring down the homophobe instead.

> I think men *are* trying to make changes. Men are themselves polic-ing inappropriate behaviours and problematic, toxic versions of masculinity. I'm not saying it's happening all the time, but I think men do that. Banter is far more complex than we often acknowl-edge. Men have ways of communicating and interacting which allow them to explore different facets of their masculinity.

This suggests that a male tribe is not a solid wall, but an active, churning mass continually competing, yes, but also correcting, chastising, or accepting. The game for any individual within it is to stay connected as it moves. This makes it highly addictive, yet fraught with unspoken anxiety: you don't want to be left out, play-ing a fruit machine alone while watching your phone screen stay dead. For young men, your group can be the primary source of your identity, but since it shifts you do need to be in the loop at all times to ensure you are performing Being A Man in the right way for your environment. And it feels good when you seem to have it right and you belong.

Without putting too fine a point on it, banter can be about making sense of failure, with the understanding that it could happen to any of us. You dish it out, but sooner or later you're going to have to take it, too. Essentially, humour is a way for men to laugh at their own pretence of being an all-powerful Real Man. Moreover, the subtleties of affection, rivalries, jealousies, attraction (though most would deny it) all exist within yobbo male groups just as much as in supposedly contrasting female groups. And guess what? There are mixed-gender groups too, providing further shifting dynamics.

Now this isn't to say that there aren't some bad eggs involved, who vindictively pull everyone down because they're so insecure about their own position. We've all met those guys. Within the ever-present all-male friendship gang it would be remiss to say emotional chat about mental health is suddenly accepted. Damien Ridge said the evidence suggested that men still meet with rejection.

Indeed, let's be honest: men can be absolute animals when they're in a group. Coming from the entitlement of a society in which men are presumed to have priority, part of the dangerous pleasure of a male gang is the mutual conspiracy of not having to care about your behaviour. At work or home you'd never say some of the things you would with your mates. It's a safe space because it's one in which you can also explore your ugly side. In fact, part of the game of 'dog' behaviour is to take it further than anyone else: to be more disgusting or outrageous. It's a hoot. A risk. Ask any man to show you the latest thread on his mates' WhatsApp group – and he won't! The buzz of giggling behind the bike sheds at ripped pages of pornography never truly leaves your system. Naughty boys forever.

Less palatable still is the thought that behaviour that might be a giggle and a lark to the group itself can be ramped up in actions aimed outwards, and all too often as intimidation: towards other male groups, and women too. The number of times my partner has returned from a night out with her friends to complain it had been ruined by a group of men who wouldn't leave them alone. Drunken leering ('What's your name, darlin'?') turning to abuse ('What, are you fuckin' frigid?'). It is important to understand male group behaviour, but equally important to draw a big line when it comes to threatening behaviour, and it shouldn't have to be left to the victims to defend themselves when there's other men standing around looking at their shoes. Not that my partner took it ('No, you're just rude. Fuck off.')

Is this our true selves coming out when given the opportunity? Or just another performance at the less savoury end of the spectrum? Enter, stage left, the 'incels'. In the online chatrooms of the Manosphere, shuffling into view in their Cannibal Corpse hoodies, these 'involuntary celibates', along with their fellow anti-feminist trolls, throw on abhorrent personae like Halloween make-up. Using extreme, misogynistic, violent language, they act like male outcasts, rejected by jocks and pretty-boys who girls swoon over (they call them 'Chads'), while resorting to the dominant clichés of masculinity: aggression, risk, heteronormativity, violence.

THREAD: Insulted by a faggot normie and a lesbian

USER 3: Back in the old days fags and dykes like them got beaten by pipes made off steal [*sic*] I don't wish harm to anyone but I honestly wouldn't give a care if these people got beaten up by a bunch of nazis they deserve it.

THREAD: Violence against girls

FEMALE USER: we need to stop this violence against girls, its just disturbing how killing girls is normalised

MALE USER: I don't care, they won't let me fuck them when they're alive.

USER 2: Women normally deservee [*sic*] it anyway

[Other user brings up a news story about a woman who killed her husband and was given custody of the child]

USER 3: But he wasn't a chad. If you are not a chad you are literally an unperson in this clown world.

USER 4: Mega retarded thread. Everyday, millions of men are killed because this or that. But guess what? Nobody cares about them because they are men. But 1 woman is killed and everuone [*sic*] lost their shit. Woman can literally kill any guy. Put some random excuse and she will be free in no time.

FEMALE USER 2: True but men are more likely to be perpetrators of violent crimes than women.

USER 3: And? Who cares? You should blame your amazing personality detector. Women love to associate with violent men.

Most of these people, you sense, are young men living at home with their parents: perfectly nice by day, but turning to the dark side at the computer at night; content to revel in an alter ego, urging each other on to say the most horrible thing they can think of. It may be just another way of acting up to the ideals of their online locations, but it's the uncomfortable face of male group banter when there are no correctives. In the US, some incels have murdered in their hate and envy.

Incels, Kitty suggested, were reasserting their masculinity. With no 'capital' to draw on from, say, sport at school, they found a space where they could demonstrate masculinity – using the same tools like aggression – in a different way. She'd coined the term 'mischievous masculinity' for the general inclination to say or do something socially unacceptable. It is a term that suggests men knowingly make such a choice, which contradicts how men and boys have been viewed in the past. 'Historically it's been: boys will be boys,' she said, 'men can't help themselves when they get together. But I argue that men have agency in a way that often isn't acknowledged. Men are actively making choices to behave in that way.' She saw the 'anything goes' male group as another post-war hangover: with economic circumstances forcing men to work all hours, a narrative had come into play whereby any free time was 'their time', as opposed to family time. To escape from the pressure of their job they were allowed to go to the pub or the rugby club to be their true selves.

As further illustration Kitty pointed me to some other sociological theories. Irving Goffman's dramaturgy theory, for example, postulates a 'front stage' – the person you are in public – and a 'back stage' – the one you are in private. The two may be very different: you will use different behavioural 'props' to display different identities. Kitty had been teaching students a theory she based upon the idea that there are many more versions of us waiting in the wings.

> Imagine we're juggling and can magically juggle a hundred balls. At certain times you're holding certain ones, and other times they're up in the air. I think a lot of the negative narratives of masculinity are just about the ones in their hands at a particular time, rather than the sum of all the parts in the air too. What's more interesting than saying men are toxic is asking: what it is about certain environments that makes men behave in those ways? That allows these accountants, lawyers, policemen, to go to a rugby club, strip naked and act like a maniac – then go home to their wife and kids?

Just because masculinity is performative does not mean it's necessarily foolish or fake: compared with the old idea of an 'authentic self' – the rugged creature we've seen in endless marketing campaigns – the idea of multiple masculinities opens up a realm of options for Being a Man. The dominant social convention at any moment, stressed Kitty in conclusion, is unstable: 'In ten years' time in this country the dominant form could be homosexuality and vulnerability. But if we could just have a masculinity that's more inclusive then we'd be laughing.'

After taking my leave of Kitty I went in to the University Arms anyway, among students with half-grown beards and half-formed dress sense. I remembered that feeling of incompleteness with fondness: the half-self was exciting in its imperfection before the working world would demand solidity. The half-self is brave, the fully formed self fearful. I caught a glimpse of a stooped man in the mirror behind the bar double-fisting two pints of strong ale: I was a fully-formed sack of shit. 'Men think there's a finished product to get to,' Kitty had said to me before I left:

> That you have a rite of passage and become a man. But what happens when you don't arrive there? Or if it happens and you can't maintain it – you lose your job, your wife, your standing? This is when men's mental health problems happen: because they've been spat out of a system that says, 'Congratulations, you're a man!' but then abandons you if you're not living up to the kind of man you're supposed to be.

What male tribes do is offer a guidebook for male behaviour, well-worn, familiar and handed down through the years. Such tribes therefore tend to be conservative and reward conformity: collectively you can vehemently resist change, because change means the perilous unknown and men are conscious of appearing strong. Nevertheless, a tribe is alert to shifts in the equilibrium, any straying from the norm: the brutal piss-taking is at least evidence of a curiosity beneath the hostility.

For a tribe radical change is somewhat uncomfortable, but change is possible, and this is where your tribe can make a difference, by picking up the pieces from the system that is chewing you all up and spitting you out again. The phenomenon of the secondary WhatsApp group offers two or three people the opportunity for meaningful chat outside the meme-filled main group. I remember speaking to a guy at the Movember Awards who had lost a mate to suicide. Now he and his mates had one group chat solely for mental health, where they had to check in regularly via a voice note, with no banter permitted. A pure, safe space in which to reveal anything. Such small adjustments could save plenty of lives.

Men need to get their heads around prevention. Bereaved friends, soldiers experiencing PTSD, addicts in recovery, prisoners in group therapy: all are examples of tribes dealing in connection and honest contemplation, without sacrificing the piss-taking. Why should you have to go through life trauma first to experience that? Especially when it holds the potential to *prevent* life traumas.

When I interviewed Joe Gilgun – best known as Woody in *This Is England* and for fictionalising his bipolar disorder in the series *Brassic* – he had a marvellous take on breaking through the intimacy barrier in male friendships.

I say this all the time: one of the biggest problems is not knowing how to talk. How the fuck *do* you talk about the way you fucking feel if you've never really done it before? But just, like, *start*! It's like the gym: no-one *wants* to do it. I don't want to do it, dude, but I have to. I fucking have to.

Cleaning up a mess is a nightmare. When you knock your Cheerios over that's a mess, and if you don't sort it out, it's going to get worse. You have to make a start. It's not enough to have a chat with your pal and sweep it under the carpet and feel good for one fucking day. People talk about mental health and being a man. In my book a fucking man sorts his shit out. Ask most women what they respect in a man, it would be that very thing. *Be vulnerable.* No-one's perfect, we're all a bunch of cunts. It's *all right*.

Joe is a prophet for our age, for what else is there but to lay yourself on the line as the absolute state you are? Only then can you start addressing things.

'Let's do it again soon,' one of my pals said, as I left the O2, and I said *Definitely*, but I knew I wouldn't. It was hard to pinpoint exactly why.

On the way home I realised that the isolation I'd inflicted on myself since losing my old job had psychologically altered me. Protective barriers had been piled up higher than they'd been in years. A hardening produced by shame. My softer masculinities had become reserved for my life at home with my partner and children; only they would see my broader spectrum. Now, I'd grown tired of giving the outside world the more restrictive public version of me. If it required the compromised version, then I'd turn away, and give it nothing at all. The self-isolation was perceived disgrace, but also disgust at what the world wanted.

Was this what people called 'masculinity in crisis'? A defeat of the spirit, a loss of faith in yourself. And how did this annihilation of values relate to the outside world?

'I don't think it's so much a crisis of masculinity,' Kitty had said to me at one point, 'so much as a crisis with what's going on in the world.' Damien Ridge had also been thinking about this.

Ever since the financial crash of 2008 I think people subconsciously realised the world isn't working as it should. The world is on fire. It is falling apart. The financial system, politics, the environment: nothing is working. Which is why you have the likes of Trump – these strongmen politicians saying everything is fine, which helps everyone stay in denial. In fact they say: let's turn up the dial on neo-liberalism and burn the world. It goes beyond gender, but gender is part of it, because these are men and it was a male-led old world. There's lots of fear. Everything is up for grabs now. We have to move into a different kind of world: it's not going to continue to work.

Everything interacts dynamically. The man exists in the tribe, which exists in the environment. And, sure as hell, if your environment sucks, your group is going to react negatively, as will you within it. Any utopian ideas of new tribes of men are going to fall pretty flat if their life experiences are filled with brutality. Men don't exist in a vacuum, and neither does masculinity: if it turns toxic it is more likely to become a rotten environment. One where the mark of a man is violence.

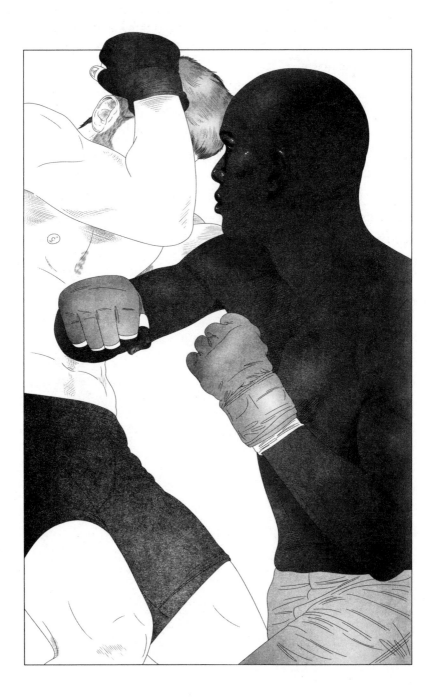

3

You Are Hard

Violence, Environment, Power

It was a miserable day in Nottingham, exactly as you'd wish given who I was there to see. Sleaford Mods' lyrical wrecking ball Jason Williamson was waiting to greet me off the train with his dole scowl, severe fringe and massive drug-dealer coat all in place. If nowadays, as he spits in 'McFlurry', 'People look like emails,' he looks more like a ransom note tied to a brick. It may be projection from knowing his songs, but the eyes seem to tell stories of a million shit jobs with a million knobheads and are ready for whatever bullshit is coming next. Not a cynic but a man with the power to look at life as it really is. I waved nervously, and he brightened.

As we walked through the centre of Nottingham, the public face of a city masking the grotty realities of Jason's territory – 'Nottz with a Z, you cunt' – it was quickly apparent that he was lovely as anything, and keen to accommodate me with somewhere peaceful to talk. Sceptics seem to think Sleaford Mods are anti-life, when in fact they have an abundance of it – too much you might say: it spills all over your shoes. Jason and his bandmate Andrew Fearn unpeel the rotten orange of life in Britain, most pointedly the post-2008 'austerity measures' by which the poor got poorer and the rich got richer and aspiration died. With Jason's obscene, hilarious, vicious rants spewing over haunted and heavy beats, they waved a sodden rag of anti-nostalgia. Listening to them was to affirm that life in this country is a rigged game: if you're from a certain class in certain regions, you can't escape. So what are you supposed to do, other than take the piss and enough drugs to make it through another shift? If anyone can give me a dose of reality when it comes to male behaviour, it's Jason.

Settled for coffee, taking on breeze blocks of cake, we talked about the famous men that first made an impression on him as a kid: Charlton Heston in *Ben-Hur*, Steve McQueen in *The Great Escape*, tormented actors like Richard Burton and Brits with regional accents like the *Carry On* crew. *Rocky* was the big one for him, both the film and the story of Stallone's struggle to get it made. 'I was obsessed with him,' said Jason. 'It really influenced me – a story of hard knocks where he'd done 500 auditions and vowed always to remember those who treated him well on the way up. But that really stayed with me: *to keep going.*'

Jason did indeed spend years trying to make it. At first he went into acting, but in the rarefied world of received pronunciation he found his class insecurities hampered him whenever he landed his 'verbal haystack'. Plus the drama school fees were prohibitive when he had a bunch of bad habits to take care of. Plan B was music: cue years in a succession of bands, moving down to London, then out to San Francisco, then back to Nottingham, all the while working crap jobs in a chicken factory and in a Little Chef, the branches of which always looked like they were hiding something, and in this case were: Jason. He was doing drugs and getting older while he tried to find something that truly worked musically.

And then he did. Someone stopped by the studio and stuck on a thrash metal CD. Jason asked the producer to loop a section and started ranting over the top.

> And that was it! With this, I could do what I wanted. I could be vulgar, I could be really bleak, and yet somehow I could bind it all up in a humorous way which carried it. It bounced. And I remember saying to a friend, 'This is it: fucking everyone is going to get it now.' He was like, 'Umm . . .' It took another ten years from that point to get anywhere.

The slow and bloody-minded crawl to the top: that's closer to the British way than the American Dream, isn't it? The Great British Grind. 'That first album [*Austerity Dogs*] was an accumulation of years of hardship and the politics of unskilled labour, shit bosses, my hatred for shit bands,' said Jason.

> It all came out. The coalition had just got in, austerity had got underway, and so it fit perfectly with that time. And that's why it was elevated, I think: we caught a period in that time. It was everything I wanted it to be. Everything I'd dreamed of, happened. Happened at 42 years of age.

The word 'masculinity' makes him wince. He feels it's used as a woke card. It's not something he's particularly gone into in his lyrics, where he's looking at people in relation to poverty, survival, dealing with what's in front of you. 'I think when it adopts an energy where it encourages you to be misogynistic,' he pondered;

> when it encourages you to be aggressive needlessly: then I've got issues with it. But there's various reasons why people don't think for themselves. Is masculinity a part of that? Probably. But there's a broader picture. And what's wrong with feeling like a man, and wanting to get buff? A lot of people haven't got a lot, apart from

a job, a little bit of money to buy things at the weekend, the gym and a vodka session after work on a Saturday. It's not the basis for advancement, but at the same time, what else have you got? What are you going to do – take yourself out of that and sit in your room?

Point taken. Easy to ask for self-analysis and explore multiple masculinities when your prospects aren't limited by an 'iron ceiling', as Jason put it. Isn't the key Truth About Men simply that we are products of our environment? If we're brought up with not much money, parental abuse, poor education, then what? How will that translate into male behaviour? Violence is picked up from the world around you. 'If someone goes out at the weekend looking for a fight you can feel it,' said Jason.

> But you should then ask yourself: why are they in that position? How do you know what they've been through? They're in that position because they're sad, feeling shit about something, something subconscious a lot of the time. And it is usually around childhood trauma, or employment situations based in the present – so is that toxic masculinity? I think it's a political issue. Also, all this is a bit classist really, let's face it. A lot of the people getting pissed and fighting are the lower-class people, so this is almost like a suppression of that existence, when that existence is a complete result of the existence above it, and the one above that.

An imperious elite creates downtrodden environments, and then blames people for acting out. The classic right-wing spread: 'Louts Cause Havoc On High Street.' The classic poverty-porn left-wing reportage: 'One Night in Scunthorpe', where all the regional dimwits in crap clothes screw each other in sticky clubs. Superior sneering from all angles.

Jason ordered more slabs of cake; he doesn't drink, do drugs or smoke any more: just coffee and cake, balanced by hardcore exercise at the gym. 'I don't like thick cunts on a Saturday in town,' he said:

> Forest lads coming home from the match in big gangs looking your wife up and down, blowing smoke in your face – there's not a lot you can do about it because there's eight lads on coke that will kick the fuck out of you. I don't like that. But again, is that masculinity? To me it is all a result of oppression, depression, circumstance and upbringing.

If masculine extremes are born out of hatred, fear, rage and humiliation, then better living conditions, better wages, better education, better mental health support should make such extremes less prevalent. 'If you look at any grime or drill music by people from poorer backgrounds,' said Jason,

> it's about getting into the world of consumerism: 'I need to sell drugs to get money to wear these clothes. Being legitimate – what's that?' You find as you go up the class scale, things get more obtainable. The idea you can get lots of money through a profession or having natural inclination for it, is information that hasn't been fed down to the bottom. To live in the world for a reason is such an alien thing to a lot of people in that situation, where it's just dog eat dog, it's fucking brutal.

Sleaford Mods' songs are not about being a man as such: more like trying to gain some dignity as a man in the absence of a decent living, or just getting off your head to deal with it, or just giving up and descending into a state of enduring loneliness where suicide might be on the cards, or not – what does it matter?

From Sleaford Mods' 'Top It Up':
Two lines on the table at a fucking funeral for somebody who got
  sick of two lines on the table

Top it up
At least the DJ's alright
I'm on a buzz
Shove it up.

Maybe the gangs of lads in the streets of this country are following the same old Being A Man guidebook, but what else can you
expect? Where are the options? Maybe they're getting through life
as best they can, with the tools at their disposal; if those tools are
of an unsavoury kind to many, it's important to understand it's
the environment which provides them. Here, 'ordinary' masculinity is not a lifestyle choice but the only thing you know. And,
faced with few prospects, is it any wonder they're trying to get basic
kicks in the absence of any opportunity to elevate themselves?

Elevate themselves? See – that's part of the problem: condescension.

What is the goal of reassessing masculinity? To 'elevate' men
to an acceptable level of bourgeois respectability? Implying
that you're some lower form of life until you have a lifestyle of
acceptable sophistication? A carefully curated presentation of bland
respectability and casual prejudice, featuring a closed network
of Identikit friends sharing horror stories of murders on nearby
estates while phoning a dealer for a cheeky after-dinner line? No,
shouldn't this be about expanding the possibilities to everyone
within their environment, not to elevate everyone to the same
middlebrow level? Seeding potential greatness on a person's own
terms? And by extension, encouraging better behaviour towards
other people, less aggro, by means of empowerment and respect?

Jason finished his second piece of cake and folded his arms,
which sported the kind of tattoos people had before tattoos
became trendy: mistakes. I looked at this complicated figure,
both unflinching recorder of 'liveable shit' and defender of that

shit from nefarious forces, and thought of an observation of James Baldwin's: 'Where there is no vision, the people perish.'

Jason left me with his conviction that it all comes back to politics.

There has to be a complete makeover of the apparatus that we live within, use, and are given. And that is a political thing. The golden days of late capitalism are over, aren't they? It has a funny way of reinventing itself, but it's made the world smaller, and made each tier in this country tighter, with fewer options. It's not just the working classes: the lower and middle classes have felt the pinch as well. There's no security around jobs, whereas the lower classes have no jobs at all. All this encourages that mindset of depression and desperation, and that's when problems arise.

No wonder violence has taken hold among young lads on estates.

What kills men? Many things. Men die earlier than women.

I was at the Engendering Men's Health conference in a busy lecture hall, and counting the number of men in the audience: seven. Seven and a half, including me. Lots of women are engaged in male matters, but the fellas, less so. Strange. Or not strange at all. The men carry on as normal, sitting in front of the TV while their house burns down, because they are in charge of the remote control and won't let it go.

Veronica Magar from the World Health Organization was on stage talking us through a report on why it is that boys born in 2008 will on average live to 68.6, and girls to 73.1. There is no biological reason for men to die younger, she told us: traditional masculinity is the problem. The mortality rate for TB around the world for men is twice that of women, which has been attributed to men not seeking treatment early enough. They tough it out, then die. Road accidents kill far more men because they take greater risks behind the wheel. Tobacco, alcohol and drugs kill far more men for the same reasons and because, well, it's a man's way to fix the problems plaguing you.

What do men kill? Many things.

Each other. In 2019, 79 per cent of worldwide homicide victims were male.

Women. 36 per cent of homicides in the UK in 2019. A rising figure.

Themselves. 75 per cent of suicides in the UK. Rising.

In all these cases, the lower the social class, the bigger share of the above statistics.

Why are men so much more violent than women? Are we born killers? While anger may be one of men's few socially acceptable expressions of emotion, violence in itself is not natural. Violence may be used in the blind heat of rage or to gain or defend power, according to the hegemonic urge, but it is not inevitable. There are other means to win status, like wit or a better coat. Neither violence nor power is a natural phenomenon, wrote the philosopher Hannah Arendt in the 1960s: 'that is, a manifestation of the life process; they belong to the political realm of human affairs whose essentially human quality is guaranteed by man's faculty of action, the ability to begin something new.' In other words, violence (and its close conspirator, power) is not natural in the way sex or eating are, but rather a consequence of human interaction and a desire to create change. That's not to sugar-coat it, merely to say that violence is dependent on who is using it, where and why. It does not follow that if you're a person – even a man! – you are violent. You are *capable* of it, but if you go without it you won't be nipping outside for a quick scrap so you can sleep.

Men of peace have been as influential in history as men of war. But if history had come at them from a different angle those men could potentially have swung either way. Indeed, any closer look usually reveals a muddied reality. Barack Obama, an honourable, intelligent man leading a relatively stable America (particularly in light of what followed), still managed to pioneer drone strikes and in 2016 drop 26,171 bombs on seven countries. Given the right circumstances, anyone is capable of picking up that tool of violence, and often – more often than we'd like – we need to act violently. The word 'violence' is tinged with evil – with reason, given the wars, torture and terrorism on the daily news cycle – but violence can also be used for revolution against oppression, protests against corruption, the instigation of political change, or defence against invaders jemmying the back door. The capability of violence, then, is not something you'd want to extinguish from humanity, not when the police murder innocent black men, and not when ISIS are torturing gay people and raping women and children. Sometimes we need to stand up and fight against injustice and terror.

Yet what about personal violence: the violence that is happening down the street? If all humans are capable of acting violently, then why, according to a WHO report, are *men* responsible for around 96 per cent of all homicides?

Part of understanding the male link to violence is to see how it is most often found among the powerful, and the powerless. The ones at the top with everything to lose, and the ones at the bottom with nothing to lose. And this is where masculinity comes into play. For men in society are assumed to be powerful. The ones in control, therefore, have a lot to lose, on a personal level aside from everything else, and the ones without control, at the bottom of the rung, want to deal with the shame that comes with it by *proving* their masculinity. In the dynamics of the male tribe, violence can implement or overturn a hierarchy, but it can also be simply a way to re-establish your credentials in the ever-vigilant policing of masculine display.

Violence takes the form of what surrounds it, the territory of the tribe shaping its expressions: knives on the street or dead arms in school. It's an effective way to perform Being a Man in front of a group (we will return to the individuals who do it behind closed doors later), due to the strong element of risk. The willingness to subject another person to pain, and put yourself in physical danger in the process, is something most would recoil from; hence its transgressive allure. The risk factor even extends to rejection from the group, if the violence is directed at the wrong person for the wrong reason. But if it is a show of strength which instils fear in others, it can create something which passes for respect, and if it represents an injustice tackled, then it may well be deemed heroic, your ticket to admiration. To lose control with the idea of gaining control. Of course, as with many of the illusions around masculinity, to lose control can mean to lose everything.

Violence may not naturally exist in you as a man, but it's an age-old way to prove you are one. Or to expose you as not much of a man at all.

'Put your phone away, you fucking prick.'

I was walking along the front in Margate in December, with the sea invisible in the dark. The words hooked into me, trying to force me to turn around. I tilted my head, that's all.

I'd been vaguely aware of the gang of lads smoking outside the bar as I passed, but they hadn't made an impression. I was floating along following directions on my phone, a disembodied mind, until those words dropped me back into my boots. A great dread inflated me to comic proportions. I was a lone man walking around on a Saturday evening before Christmas getting called out by the traditional gang of amateur drinkers trying to out-dick one another. I knew what I had to do. Nothing.

I ignored the jeers, thought of rainbows and unicorns, muttered 'Cunts' under my breath and hurried on without hurrying.

Was it fucking prickish to be holding my phone to my face as I walked? To be following this ridiculous nagging green arrow out of habit more than need? – I could see the chip shop up ahead anyway. I put my phone back in my pocket.

'Wa-haay!'

'Pussy!'

'Queer boy!'

'What a fucking pussy!"

Oh, I do like to be beside the seaside.

Don't react, don't give them anything.

My partner and kids were waiting inside the Airbnb for their tea. I gave the whole cacophony behind me The Shrug Off. *I came of age in the squaddie pubs of Beverley, lads. Avoiding fights is in the blood.*

In the chip shop I watched the boiling fat bubble and spit. When I was handed my order the girl was chatting to me but I couldn't hear what she was saying. Back outside, the inconsolable sea smacked its head repeatedly into a wall out in the void. I bought a cheap bottle of wine from a corner shop and started picking the price label off as I walked so my partner wouldn't know how cheap it was.

Around the dining table in the flat we were all eating the chips out of the paper and watching Ant and Dec on the TV. My kids love these kind of family treats. Me too, usually, but I was elsewhere.

In my head I was playing reels of action:

'You fucking cunts, come on then, come on, I'll fucking kill you'
get your keys between your fingers
sneak in the back way, buy a bottle, smash it into one of their heads
thumbs gouging into eye sockets, don't stop till they drag you off

'Are you OK?' asked Marian.

I'm fine.

I smiled, flushing. This was a chance to show I was getting better at saying what was on my mind. I told her what happened, and then I told her that I was going back out to beat the men up. I was serious, until I saw her face.

Still, I couldn't sleep that night. I turned over and over in humiliation. The lads, in their safe little group, had shamed me. And I took it. Like always.

What could I have done? They'd probably – inevitably – have kicked my head into the kerb. I couldn't have eaten my chips with my kids if I was brain-damaged.

I'm not a fighter. I'm not tough, and I do find it embarrassing. I've always been tall but physically weak. A Giacometti sculpture made of Marmite. The kind of sap who'd reference Giacometti. If only I was stacked: then I'd carry myself differently and, if not actively search for fights, at least know I could handle myself.

This tied into an anxiety about my weakness as a man. When you are adept at invisibility you can generally avoid being tested out. But as had happened many times before, I felt my nerves twitching with a desire to inflict physical punishment on such idiots. I found myself fantasising about violence, having never truly tried out my capacity for it. It started seeping out into my real behaviour. Road rage behind the wheel. Snapping at strangers in my way. Nursing personal slights by friends. Winding myself up to prove myself as a man. It was coming.

Part of it was linked to being a dad: could I protect my family if I needed to? Well, if required, I simply would. But what if I was overwhelmed? Beaten down; left helpless to do anything more?

It was after this episode that I started looking for a gym to work out. I said to myself, *I'm doing it for my family.* Like Walter White from *Breaking Bad*. As with him, my actual motivation was about ego. I wanted power. To feel like a man.

'Less than. I felt less than.'

Jamie dipped his biscuit, leaned forward, pleased to talk it through, it seemed. It was a brutal winter's day, and through the window the wind could be seen whipping people back inside the buildings. Only the giant oaks were bearing up against it, shaking off a few dead branches. It may have looked like a college campus, but it didn't feel like one. HMP Spring Hill is a Category D men's prison in Buckinghamshire, a transitional place for low-risk inmates to start to find work, receive counselling and get back into society. Jamie and I were sat in the office of the DART (Drug and Alcohol Recovery Team) staff, and he was telling me about the pressures he felt as a man growing up on an estate in Hounslow, West London.

'I got into this life because of identity,' he said. 'I felt less than when I was young. I used to feel like I wasn't the toughest in my area. I felt like a pushover, and I didn't want to be like that. I wanted to be like the men in the pub.'

Jamie's current stretch is seven years, his longest. Having grown up with a need to prove his worth as a young man he eventually ran smack into the full weight of macho behaviour at Wormwood Scrubs: 'In there it really is about who's biggest, hardest, most violent.' Now he's finally come to conclusion that it's 'all bollocks'.

Less than. He told me more about how the feeling always played upon him. He was a small kid, and wasn't the most confident. He was adrift, had mental health issues; his mum was tough but his dad generally absent and unimpressive when present. Not like the men Jamie loved in *The Sopranos*, and not like the men down the pub. He lacked guidance, people to talk to, a place to be accepted.

The pub provided what was missing, but led him into all kinds of 'madness'.

'Men do "man up" in front of each other,' he said.

> Constantly. I remember the first time I was properly violent. We were sat in the pub, and there was this bloke there. My mate, who I looked up to, said, 'Go on, Jamie, do him.' I didn't want to, but I was put on the spot, and I didn't want to feel like an idiot. So I hit him with a glass. I was always trying to prove myself to the people I was hanging out with.

Goodfellas. That was the film that did it for him. 'As far back as I can remember, I always wanted to be a gangster.' He wanted that: *to be someone.* The men he met at the pub granted him access to that crime world, and there he felt as though he belonged, even though he was obviously exploited: 'You're only as good as the last bit of money you earned.' He even felt his closest mates were just using him. Still, if the camaraderie was imagined the drink and the drugs made it *feel* real. 'You trusted each other,' he recalled. 'You had each other's back, no matter what madness happened. Misplaced loyalty.'

Now Jamie's been through a system of mental health support inside he's come to understand that something had been wrong all that time. Depression and bipolar. Back then he couldn't talk about those stresses, though. He'd hide any vulnerabilities from the crowd he'd become part of, not wanting to risk his position in the group. 'When I was alone I'd worry if anyone liked me. "Why aren't they calling me?" I worried they didn't give a shit, that I was an outcast, a misfit.' His way of showing them that he was worthy of being one of them was by being 'a little bastard'. He didn't know who he was, had no identity, but thought he could find one through their eyes. When he was among them it all came together, helped by the drugs, and the days became addictive in many different ways: 'Wake up with nothing, go out to rob shops, nick clothes, sell them, buy drugs, meet up, go out fighting, meet some girls, enjoy the buzz, breaking all the rules. Start all over again the next morning. Better than a nine-to-five.'

More damaging too, and there was always a lot to prove. Jamie liked to hang with the hardest men, and since his size meant he was never going to be physically dominant he earned his respect by being the most violent. He started carrying a knife. It coincided with him deteriorating mentally. 'I felt trapped in my own head. It all came out one night.' In a confrontation, he stabbed someone, and that was the end of that. Except it wasn't.

'Even in prison it didn't stop,' he said, 'I was twenty-six, twenty-seven, but I sought out the hardest inmates. The top men. I always wanted to be with the baddest ones. My identity was so lacking I was looking for people to follow. It just meant more madness. You can get anything you want in prison.'

Gradually, however, he began turning himself around. Now he was in Narcotics Anonymous, recovering, taking stock, and seemed well liked by the DART team, able to analyse himself with good humour. When he leaves Spring Hill he has the intention of being a good dad to his kid: 'I know I'm not a bad person. I made some bad decisions, but I was a product of my environment.' He's dealing with the mental health issues, his bipolar, and thinks there's still time for him to achieve. He wants to be loved, and thinks people can change. He knows it's going to be hard to shake his past, but he hopes his age and experience will now help. Still, it will be hard to shed the past and the old feelings. 'I was out in Oxford with my daughter, looking about at all these normal people and I thought . . . this is nothing. What a boring life.'

Back at the Engendering Men's Health conference, Gary Barker, the CEO of Promundo (an organization which works with boys and men around the world to promote gender equality and prevent violence), was guiding us through a study of men in the US, UK and Mexico called 'The Man Box'. The results showed that men felt they had to prove their worth *as* men with violent behaviour. Particularly *in front of* other men. It's a route to group acceptance, personal respect and identity, but which creates chains of destructive behaviour. Forty-one per cent of men in the UK agreed that 'A man who doesn't fight back when others push him around is weak.'

This need to prove your masculinity when it is questioned goes to the heart of many problems with men. That's your gang warfare right there, plus your global warfare by statesmen snubbed at NATO conferences. The need for respect is paramount – but what is respect? A gift given when a person reaches a certain admirable position, a fulfilment of the hegemonic ideal in your environment. Respect must therefore be earned in the eyes of others. And in the maelstrom of male groups it must be performed again and again, for respect is also something which can be whipped away from you at any moment: a pratfall spilling pints, a spooned open goal, cowardice in the face of a fight. As we've seen, humour will cover a multitude of embarrassments, but serious disrespect, a questioning of status with intent, particularly by someone outside the core group, demands a more overt action to restore your standing. A 'word'. A fight. Worse.

With violence so present in the mind if not the hands of groups, it raises another question about violence: do people enjoy it? If people are products of their environment, and their environment is filled with violence, then using violence must come with psychological rewards. Not to mention physiological ones: the adrenaline of contact, the dopamine rush if you escape in better shape than the other guy. The mythic rewards too: the fulfilment of the warrior ideal fed into your head via popular culture thrills – for one moment you *were* Jason Bourne, even if the reality was scuffling in sodden exhaustion beneath a urinal.

The thrill of it is there, and what a dark one it is too, because it is uncontrolled. One of you could end up dead. Given the size of your average gym bunny these days, it's no surprise that we are in the era of 'one-punch deaths'. The readiness to hurt is disturbing. As is the role of spectators, your tribe being the immediate respondents, your prime audience of critics, taking notes. Likely strangers want to watch the violence too. Pub rubberneckers eager to see the worst to have a grisly story to tell about their night out. Everyone fascinated to see who might win in this race to the bottom. The contest and the horror of it. Violent thrills on a night out for the working class, violent thrills on a night in for the middle classes; screens full of violence providing some titillation for those sitting on plump sofas. Transgressive fantasies to gawp at with a bowl of luxury ice cream melting in your lap. Doesn't everyone love violence in some form?

Smack, twist, squeeze.

You can civilize yourself to the point where you exfoliate your scrotum, but the fascination with humans pummelling each other in tiny shorts never really goes away.

Grunt, snort, grind.

Two men were wrapped around each other in the Octagon ring. It was hard to see exactly what was going on, as they were locked on the floor in a sweaty smear of body parts. First one of them appeared to be trying to lock in a choke hold, then the other, but slowly, very slowly. It was a question of exhausting your opponent until you could finish them off. I'm sure it was very technical, but to me it just looked like two boa constrictors fucking.

I sipped my beer placidly in the midst of a crowd who were busy tossing theirs. This was the headline fight, Webb vs Frederick, the big moment for everyone in this venue, but only another in a long night of fights for us cage-fighting virgins; another chance to watch two men Kama Sutra each other to death. Beside me the Hungarian illustrator Berta Vallo was being chatted up by yet another drunken Englishman. I'd invited her along to help with the illustrations adorning this book without quite realising what we were in for. All night long I'd been apologising for the coked- and pilled-up gangs of lads stumbling into her, and the blood bursting across the Octagon, to which she'd consistently responded: 'Shut up.' Berta was having a great time getting into confrontations, refusing to move an inch for the toe-treaders, pushing them out of the way and calling them 'fucking cunts'. Since she was a rarity at the cage fighting – a woman, for a start, and one dressed like Marilyn Manson's little sister – the sight of her seemed to confuse the addled men, who always dutifully apologized and moved out of the way. Now she beckoned the drunk guy down to her 5-foot-3 level, and said something into his ear. He turned away quickly, ashen. Berta laughed. I didn't ask. Most of my night had been spent pretending not to be with her. Only one of us was going to end up getting punched, and it wasn't Berta.

A roar went up. The two men in the Octagon had separated and Frederick was slamming enormous haymakers at Webb's head, connecting over and over until Webb slumped, unable to defend himself. The ref stepped between them, waving extravagant arm Xs. It was over.

As if cued, the action suddenly transferred from the stage to the floor of the venue. Frederick's Birmingham contingent suddenly rushed into Webb's supporters from Essex, who until that point had been dominating the arena. In the semi-darkness the men seemed to collapse in on each other and liquify.

We were standing a couple of metres away, too close. *Let's get out of here*, I said to Berta. She seemed to think about it for a second, then slowly, calmly, as in a sickening dream, walked straight forward into the thick of the ruck.

What are you doing? I yelled in a panic, reaching for her as I'd reach for my falling child at soft play, but she was gone.

It was chaos. Charging bodies, grimacing faces, a lunatic giggling as he slipped to the floor and stayed there on his back. Bloodied men were being led out of the ruck by furious girlfriends or huge security guards. Frederick was on the edge of the stage, asking for calm but with a smile on his face, his eyes still glittering from victory.

At last Berta popped out from somewhere along the east face of the swarm, heading back towards me, grinning.

Come on, let's get out of here.

'No, I want to watch. This is so funny.'

You're going to get hurt.

'I'm fine, shut up.'

Look, I'm a dad, I just want to . . . what, protect her? Or protect myself? For a moment I did contemplate crouching down behind her, but was concerned my coat would dip into the river of beer and blood on the floor, so instead persuaded her to check out the merch stand.

Cage fighting is a brutal sport, one I cannot stop watching. From highlights reels it appears to be boxing on crack, but watching the fights live tonight I'd realised it's boxing on Xanax. Explosions of heavy punches and flying knees do break out, but the vast majority of the action is an embrace of attrition. It looks almost tender from a distance, one misplaced finger away from turning into heavy petting. Grunt, grind, sweat, grunt, on it goes for long five-minute rounds while the crowd crane to see what's going on. You turn up for *Fast & The Furious 6* and get Tarkovsky's *Stalker*.

Cage fighting is much closer to real-life street fights than boxing and, with its lawless undertones, has become big business, with UFC (Ultimate Fighting Championship) worth £5.7 billion, and smaller organizations in the UK, like tonight's Cage Warriors, selling out arenas, bagging TV deals and making stars out of the fighters. Naturally there has also been an attendant rise in 'white-collar' cage fighting – charity matches for amateur office workers – so everyone can get a piece of the action. Is it sport or is it violence? If it was sport on stage and violence off stage then is the distinction simply lighting? Of course it *is* a sport – the fighters were serious athletes, so built they could use me as a resistance band – but the fascination with it is rooted in how it hits all those facets of hegemonic masculinity: physical power, dominance, bravado, warrior myths and violence. It is men *in excelsis*. Yet female cage fighting is massive too, and, hell, my companion was having the time of her life; humans are drawn to this kind of spectacle. Sport as exorcism is hardly breaking news, but cage fighting presents it vividly afresh. The violence leaves you buzzing.

We bought all the merch they had and left. It struck me that for all the fighting, the most fearless thing I saw in there was Berta standing her ground.

'Web-by, Web-by, Web-by … walking in a Webby wonderland …' the venue was emptying behind us and the bloodied supporters were singing again as they roamed the O2. Always nice to be back there again. We watched as men still clutching plastic pint glasses stumbled into imitation pot plants, alarming the wine-sippers outside All Bar One, who pulled their giant GAP bags in closer.

With unfortunate timing, the Little Mix crowd were also emptying out of the main arena. At the sight of large men staggering towards them in ripped shirts, herds of young girls began running for their parents' cars. Left alone, triumphant in some obscure way, the cage-fighting fans sang under the giant LED screens previewing next week's attractions. Another successful Friday night at the country's top entertainment megaplex.

Evolutionary psychologists view violence as an inevitable consequence of being primates. Males are more prone to aggression because of sexual competition, being guardians of the territory or protecting the group from predators. Men's anatomy has evolved to reflect this, with on average 75 per cent more muscle mass than women and, in general, heavier bones, shorter reaction times, bigger lungs and thicker skin. We're primed not just for hierarchal challenge but outright combat. According to Evolutionary Neuroandrogenic Theory, male sex hormones, primarily testosterone, are correlated with males searching for resources, social position and sexual partners; because these are highly competitive fields, those hormones are therefore linked to criminality and violence. This is disputed territory, though: the endocrinologist Dr Richard Quinton told me that 'there's no evidence at all of criminality linked to testosterone,' and suggested high testosterone in Alphas at the apex of human hierarchies 'is probably due more to effect than cause . . . When the Alpha is removed, the levels of the others will go up.'

To me, this physical adaptation for violence plays a secondary role. It is only resorted to because of conflict that arises out of other human interactions, rather than from a compulsion to violence itself. Inevitably, then, some of those more outwardly manly physical traits are for display rather than action, particularly now there are fewer sabre-toothed tigers sniffing around. And while male bodies may theoretically be built for violence, one look at my friendship group would suggest a different story. Almost every man I know, including myself, looks like something dug out of the ground: wriggly, white and half-blind in daylight. Maybe it's an English thing, but until the recent fitness boom the only person you saw with a ripped body was the Jolly Green Giant. For men like us, sexual display or territorial protection becomes a matter of jokes, hair and absurd dress codes. Violence may be latent in all men, but it is environment which dictates whether it is the first tool you reach for. It is not the result of being biologically male. Indeed, the spurs to violence are often not physical threat or sexual display – not of the body at all, but of the mind; when a man's masculinity is undermined. Could it be then, that if masculinity can be unwound from its tightly coiled state, violence in society will reduce?

The Canadian evolutionary psychologists Martin Daily and Margo Wilson analysed data about murders in 14 countries, including primitive societies, and found that on average men killed 26 times more frequently than women. In the UK, though homicides in 2019 were down for the first time in five years, homicides in London rose for the third year straight, and men in their twenties were by far the biggest group of victims, with 132 men aged 20–29. Gang culture was one of the key contributors, deaths in inner cities reaching all-time highs, with schoolboys slain nightly on the streets. Is this socialized behaviour from peers and their territory, or just what happens to boys when given the right/wrong amount of freedom?

I'd talked to Professor Robin Dunbar, the evolutionary psychologist, about the role of risk within violence, and how its urges might be linked to a different kind of performance: attracting a mate.

'Risk-taking is a form of mate advertising for men,' he told me.

We did a study once looking at when males crossed at a zebra crossing against the lights, and it depended critically on whether there were women on one side of the road or the other. The women didn't take risks by and large, but the men did, and they were much more likely to do so if they had a female audience watching. Then they would dash across in front of an oncoming car. This leads to all kinds of high-risk behaviours which carry serious mortality risks. Boys are much more likely to die in their teenage years than girls are. Much more likely.

We've examined male groups in isolation, but of course they exist in a broader sense, and attracting sexual partners is all part of the buzz. Robin saw the display of violence as another form of peacocking, even in the grim slayings of knife crime. 'Essentially what this is doing is showing what good quality genes you have,' he said,

and there is no point in taking risks unless you are serious, since that's what separates the men from the boys. There's no point in playing tiddlywinks here. Putting your life on the line is a very characteristic phenomenon, where they test their physical ability and therefore their genetic superiority. Because that's what girls are looking for. Girls are attracted to naughty boys because they're the ones who have essentially demonstrated the quality of their genes.

Whether 'All girls love a bad boy' is quite how this works, I'm not sure. You could imagine group hierarchy dictating that the most admired men would be most admired by prospective sexual partners too. But do all women love a murderer? Feels like a stretch. The area of primate comparisons always makes me wary – sorry for stating the obvious, but we are not apes – but even within that field, female chimpanzees have shown preferences for Alphas who care about young ones. Male owl monkeys carry, groom, provide for and play with offspring, as well as protect. Even our hairy cousins don't agree that 'Chicks dig nutters.'

In fact, what about the real nutters? The ones who scare everyone else, who do the very worst, who take things too far? Is it not these people doing most of the damage, dragging everyone else down with them? Who hasn't been in a group of mates who have collectively cringed as one of them turns into a headcase? Robin explained the role such people play in society, and why the extreme end of male behaviour is impossible to get rid of:

> There is a tail end of male behaviour which borders on the psychopathic. How much it comes out will depend on circumstances and upbringing, but basically these guys cannot control their behaviour. They will steal from people and beat people up without being too fussed about it, and abuse women – it's all part of the same thing. They can empathize with other people but they can't sympathize with them. That's what makes them so dangerous – because they know exactly how to twist the knife to hurt you psychologically or otherwise, but they don't care.

This lot have been part of all societies, said Robin, and for useful historical reasons. 'When you went raiding on the shores of England in a longboat it was jolly good to have a couple of these guys in your boat with double-headed blood axes – all the Saxons would run off. But at home they were a complete liability.' Robin stressed that they're a small fraction of the population, but in the right circumstances they can be influential. 'You see this in something like ISIS, with civil breakdown, civil war conditions. When the rule of law is lost, then these guys come out of the woodwork, fighting with enthusiasm.'

Even more troubling is that we kind of admire other men with psychopathic tendencies. Not serial killers, but two steps removed:

the maniacs we know from football teams, workplaces, the pub. In the right arena they can be valuable allies on our metaphorical longboats, but you wouldn't want them dating your sister. One of the reasons why they are secretly, or not so secretly, admired is because they exhibit a hyper-masculinity, will take more risks than anyone. You sense you're either friends with them, or their enemies.

The question remains: how can the nutters be stopped? It may be impossible to be rid of them, but surely within the tribe men can do something about it? This question of agency: can we agree that we do possess enough intellect, if we choose to apply it, and perhaps stop more people getting killed? We can't remove violence altogether, but surely we can try to remove it as a mark of machismo?

Violence spreads like blood on a pavement. One kid gets stabbed, revenge occurs, and then you have a new standard to meet if you want to be the baddest on the block. Soon the division between the psychos and the nice kids gets blurred, and gangs are playing 'spin the gun' to see who's going to shoot the next random on the street. It is a mode of asserting who you are within a context. Agency. Violence is a membership card.

'I thought I was a pirate.' Ben, fresh out of prison, was serious. 'That's how I perceived myself. I'll do what I want to do. Drug dealing, playing with guns, not paying any taxes, not working a fucking nine-to-five. My dad was a mundane nine-to-fiver, and that was never in my plans. My idols were villainous-type people.'

Ben was on the phone to me a couple of weeks after being released from HMP Spring Hill, where I'd previously met Jamie. Now Ben was adjusting to life on the outside, with the intention of starting his own gym business. He'd served two and a half years of a five-year sentence for armed robbery. While inside he took it upon himself to address his issues. Stayed clear of the addicts on crack and heroin, and bagged a job in the gym, picking up a couple of PT qualifications and sticking with the business-minded people, the fitness freaks, the ones 'at the top of the food chain'. More importantly, when he was moved to Spring Hill and worked with the DART team, he managed to get a proper diagnosis of his mental health problems.

'I was trying to get help before I went to prison, but I was selling and sniffing cocaine because it was always around me,' he said. 'I spent most of my life in a pub environment. They couldn't properly diagnose my mental health issues because I was actively using. When I got to D Cat I was told I had Borderline Personality Disorder. Probably bipolar too, which can happen, particularly if your upbringing has been difficult.'

Ben's a south Londoner, born in Waterloo and brought up in Pimlico, then Morden. His younger brother, who's still inside, has paranoid schizophrenia. An uncle also had paranoid schizophrenia and killed himself. His mum's psychopathic disorder made her incapable of displaying emotion or showing her children any love. Consequently, aged 14 and kicked out of school, he became mixed up in gang culture with his friends, who were mostly Jamaican. While he was of mixed-race heritage, he'd experienced some of the racism directed at his peers and shared a sense of exclusion from society. He revelled in this alternative world.

I got involved in guns and the distribution of drugs, and that's where I found my comfort. Peculiar, I know, but that's what it was. I was happy around these people. Now I know it was fake love, I was just money-making for them, really, and they were older people grooming younger people, but at that point in my life I needed a family network. I thought I was a little bad boy, you know?

Big house, cars, women, money. That was what he had in mind at the start: not the nitty-gritty, the violence, the mayhem that followed. It was extreme. In a funny sort of way his BPD worked for him, he told me, because his personality is one of extremes too. He's either very low or very high. It helped in that business and it helped inside – 'You either sink or swim in prison, and I'm a swimmer.' Adapt and overcome. There was a lot to overcome: 'I've seen people die in prison, I've seen people stabbed in prison, get slashed in prison, get beaten up in prison, seen vulnerable people get raped in prison. There's no control in there.'

Now it was about opening up the gym business, and seeing how he could help younger people with their mental health issues by getting them involved in exercise. He'd also been offered a job at HMP Aylesbury mentoring young offenders from gangs serving life sentences:

> They've obviously killed someone, they've been lifed off. Now they're thinking 'What the fuck?', with the realisation they're going to be in prison for the rest of their lives, or 30 years of it, before they have a chance of parole. I want to help other people. And I want younger people to know gang life is bullshit.

Want to see some real toxic masculinity? Head to prison. While some have talked about this as the ultimate sign of what men do when they're in an exclusively male group, it's more about what happens when the environment is appalling. Over the past five years the proportion of prisoners developing a drug problem *inside* prison has doubled. In 2018/2019 the prisons watchdog said self-harm levels were 'disturbingly high' and suicides surged by 23 per cent. Since 1990 the prison population in England and Wales has doubled. Sentences are longer, in 2019 48 per cent were over four years, compared to 33 per cent in 2010. According to the Ministry of Justice 62 per cent of prisons in England and Wales were overcrowded. Is the state of male prisons a masculinity problem or a political problem? Or both?

Despite his disgust with the prison system, it had clearly given Ben a chance to reassess his life, and the work he was embarking on suggested not just that redemption is there for people who want it, but that violence can be excised from your life. That is, if you remove yourself from your environment – Ben had headed out to Devon – and escape not just the gang life but the gang mentality.

Psychopaths exist in society – will always exist, according to Robin – but what of all the other people who become caught up in criminality because of where they happened to pop into the world? Are all these criminals psychopaths, or indeed 'evil'?

It is surely a question of education; of who's stepping in to raise vulnerable young men. The elders in gangs appear to provide the role models absent elsewhere. Perhaps some of the remedy is therefore in providing better education in poorer areas, and more visible role models too. In an interview about knife crime, the rapper Wretch 32 made a plea for collective responsibility. 'We're all pointing fingers so much,' he said, 'but that's not the point. The point is we all play our part, so let's play that part . . . There is not one solution. It takes a village to raise a child – I think we have to be conscious of what part we're playing in that village.' To this end he'd made a point of staying in Tottenham, his home neighbourhood: 'If you become successful you disappear. Get as far away as possible. [Instead you should] become successful and do things in the community. Make sure you are present, and that kids see the success story as well as the negative narrative.'

Making violence on the street of the UK into a story about 'bad kids', as many politicians and media outlets do, shirks responsibility. Smacks of racism too. Of contempt for people who are deemed Other, a deviant from the nice, white Norm. Hostility is directed at all the working classes, but the worst is directed at those of 'different' colour, immigrants or refugees: those who 'don't belong here', and are thus kept on the outskirts of society. As Jason Williamson said, it's about politics. Punishment is easier and cheaper than prevention; makes for macho 'strong on crime' headlines too. But if you remove hope from an area, what's going to happen?

Meaningful funding for prevention organizations is needed, but frankly anything would be better than the current plan to simply throw more children in prison. The non-white population of the country is over-represented in prison: 27 per cent of inmates are from ethnic minorities, though they only make up 13 per cent of the general population. It doesn't take much hard work to figure out why: institutional racism and destitution. The poverty rate for BAME groups is almost twice that for whites. Poverty. Isolation. No future. What are you going to do as a young man looking for a purpose? Who's looking out for you?

Well, men like Wretch 32. None of this is hopeless.

It needs state support, but it also requires a recognition from older people – no, scratch that, older *men*, who don't particularly think it's anything to do with them – that they have a responsibility to the youngsters in their orbit to educate them in the world. The unwanted extremes of masculinity can only be countered with positive alternative forms of expression.

Because, here's the thing: *boys are fragile!*

All children are fragile, and boys are no exception. Few accept this beyond a certain age. We expect our boys to be men by the time they outgrow the cute stage and grow gawky: that they stop crying, pull themselves together, and just deal with life without complaint. This gives a vivid lesson to a vulnerable mind that they're not going to be looked after any more and now have to handle the world alone. When they don't know how. Panic can set in, a feeling a weakness, of not being like other boys, of not living up to what your father figure wants, which only reinforces the need to put on a front. If a certain toughness is what's expected of them, then existence becomes about emotional control. You'll do anything not to betray your vulnerable, naïve inner self, even though in later life this will have consequences for everything from sex to work to mental health. Boys don't have their innocence taken from them: they are forced to give it away.

Boys are fragile and can't just be abandoned. If they are, they'll be educated by their peers, schooled in playground misinformation and vacuous, vicious fantasy. If they are not looked after, supported, talked to, confided in, shown real love, then they're left with no sense of self, no worth, no innate confidence. Left to construct a shell for appearance's sake, inside which they are alone. Not all boys, but many, many boys are taught to live a lie. Not a small lie either, but a lie about their very identities.

No wonder, then, there's all this chaos. This unhappiness, this suppressed need to talk, this rage and violence, this hollowness. And no wonder there's such a discrepancy between men supposedly being in control of society, and actually feeling barely in control of themselves. No wonder, too, that extremist groups which plan atrocities against innocent people deliberately play upon this disenfranchisement and alienation by putting a masculine arm around the lost.

'What radicalizes a man, in my experience, is the question of identity, the question of belonging.' Fatima Zaman runs a Kofi Annan

Foundation Initiative called 'Extremely Together' which works to combat violent extremism. We talked on the phone. 'When you're in a situation where you feel like you don't belong', she told me,

> you can have a recruiter for an extremist organization saying, 'Here's a space where you belong. Here's a space with a position, where you can be a leader, a warrior, in a brotherhood.' They have an ideology, a narrative to follow, and they really plan it all out carefully to get their hooks into people when they're having that identity crisis.

Extremist groups don't just happen by accident, according to Fatima; they recruit, they plan, they identify who to target. And those under 30 are disproportionally affected by violent extremism, both as perpetrators and victims, as they're the ones still undergoing the formation of their identity: they can be vulnerable and impressionable, and have an absence of positive influences. It's remarkably easy to get into their minds with an ideology, she went on, and bit by bit introduce violent elements. If you're a young British Muslim man, you may still be trying to figure out how those two identities fit together. Extremists tell such individuals that they're diametrically opposed. 'It doesn't start with, "Here's an AK-47, go shoot someone,"' said Fatima,

> which is what a lot of people think. It's about ideology and narrative. It's the same with white supremacists: it's really about understanding what that individual is missing. Isolating them away and then introducing violent ideology – that usually comes third or fourth in the radicalisation process.

Fatima works all around the world, but particularly in the UK and Europe, to combat all forms of violent extremism. Uniquely, her

103

initiative works with young people, using them in a peer-to-peer approach as peace bringers to combat the very factors that threaten them. It's about prevention: helping them stay away from extremist ideology, but also working with people who have crossed the threshold and want to come out. Fatima was employed by the late Ghanaian diplomat and UN Secretary-General Kofi Annan when she was 23, and is continuing his work: 'His values about pluralism, tolerance, fairness, and equality amongst people who, because of certain societal constructs, feel like they're on opposite ends of the spectrum, and who feel they need to be violent towards one another.' Her approach, then, is not about demonizing parts of the population, but understanding them.

> The way you radicalize men and women is different, but there are similar elements around identity. Young women who don't feel like they belong, who look different, and who need a friend: that friend may say, 'Have you thought about this?' There's a sense of sisterhood. On the male side it's about being part of the gang, a friendship group with camaraderie. And then suddenly it takes you off to Syria, or getting an offensive tattoo to be a part of a white supremacist organisation.

Fatima became invested in this world after the 7/7 attacks in London. The attack outraged her and the aftermath, in which large sections of the media demonized Muslims, disturbed her. While at a local level she saw people coming together in solidarity, and was herself a member of Muslim groups talking about their identities and radicalism, nationally it seemed the talk was of Muslims being the problem.

> However, quickly I realized I didn't have to become an extremist apologist, because it wasn't my Muslim faith that was responsible. Horrific violent individuals hijacked my faith, which

was predominantly peaceful, to rain down terror on my fellow Londoners. But as I was trying process my emotions I saw a lot of friends, particularly my male friends, becoming very angry. And it hardened them. It hardened them to an extent where they became anti-state, anti-anything, because they felt they had to put up a defence mechanism. While that was a completely rational thing to a certain extent, there was a small pocket who became radicalized. In a way the extremists won twice. Not only did they hurt Britain, but the lasting legacy is continued radicalization of young men in the UK. Actually they won three times, because on the flipside you had British men of white heritage becoming radicalized too.

An important development in Fatima's field in the last few years has been the link between hyper-masculinity and violent extremism. She points to the gunman in New Zealand who live-streamed himself gunning down people in a Christchurch mosque: 'For me the question is not only what happened to him, and what was the impetus to carry out such a horrific attack, but why did he want to film it? To display such violence?'

'Strong men do not get ethnically replaced or allow their culture to degrade,' the gunman himself had written in his manifesto; 'weak men have created this situation and strong men are needed to fix it.'

'As a society we have OKed this kind of masculinity,' reflected Fatima:

the idea that a man is a man when he is powerful, and the boss, and sometimes violent, and the idea of patriarchal rule – this all feeds into the extreme end with someone like the Christchurch shooter, who believes a strong man is above everyone else and can right the wrongs as he sees fit.

You can see it with white nationalist groups in England: the wounded rage of men dimly believing they should be superior to anyone else, powerful and unquestioned. They weaponize classic male signifiers like drinking and football, egging each other on and proving their masculinity, how hard they are – the same kind of posturing Fatima said she's seen in ISIS propaganda, 'where it's all about these guys with biceps and AK-47s, posing, putting forward this extreme masculine vision of a warrior, a soldier.'

How we are raising boys and men therefore becomes a question of making the world a safer place, and masculinity nothing less than a battleground for the future. 'I do think it's difficult to be a young man in the twenty-first century,' said Fatima.

> Masculinities differ across cultural, geographical, political contexts, but there's usually a dominant and normative form of masculinity upheld by society. It conditions our men to adhere to these cultural norms, and means if you do want to be a bit sensitive, or seen as an advocate for equality, you're not a proper man. I find that disturbing, because that is a suppression of a young man.

Fatima told me how in Nigeria the militant Islamic group Boko Haram uses rape and the abduction of women not just to terrorize society, but also, as an extreme manifestation of masculinity, to radicalize its male recruits. Same with the far-right groups on the rise in Europe, where violence against women is used to 'cement that toxic masculinity which helps embed that ideology further for men'.

As Fatima stressed, it is important to recognize that, compared to other parts of the world, the UK is a relatively tolerant place, and doing better than many at integration. Nevertheless, there is much work to be done and, as society becomes more splintered in online discourse, more polarized than ever, there is a need to protect people from nefarious forces trying to take advantage of alienation and disenfranchisement. Fatima sees guided discussions around identity in schools as crucial to prevent boys exploring identities online, which may lead them to extreme content, and ultimately down extreme routes. Families taking responsibility and offering support is key. And when 'certain individuals in certain positions of power espouse a rhetoric akin to extremist organizations,' said Fatima, positive versions of masculinity need to be prominent in society. 'You're seeing things being taken back 10 or 15 years by bringing divisive views going on below the surface into the mainstream again. It's important we challenge that, and speak truth to power.'

Violence can be part of the conditioning process of becoming a man. To accept this is not to excuse it, but to try and understand it. In some cases, most obviously the armed forces, the capacity for violence is a necessary part of the role, which must be trained up as far as it can while still being under control. A civilian army of men is also being trained in violence, however, the blank-eyed, massed ranks of which are demonstrating it on the streets under the watchful eyes of elders or friendship groups. Beneath the layers of protection boys build up around themselves, they can reach for a weapon that will cut through any doubt about their masculinity. The ultimate performance.

Still, the majority of men manage to pull back from madness. Today many are doing it by taking charge of their own physical health. Establishing agency over their bodies suggests a desire to take agency over their entire lives. Building themselves into giants could be a means to tackle the colossus of masculinity inside their own heads.

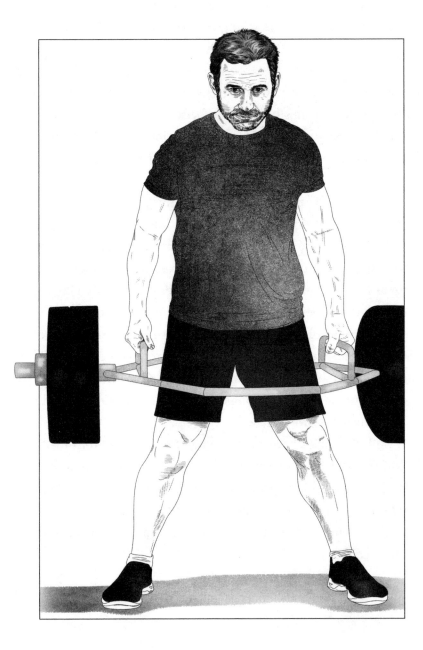

4

You Are Ripped

Fitness, Physical Heroes and the Body

The package arrived early one Saturday morning: the kind you sneak into the house while nobody's looking. The children were in front of the TV and my partner, Marian, was still in bed. I had to grab the moment.

In the kitchen, I swiftly took a knife to the package. Inside was a little blue box. I pulled it open and emptied the contents onto the table. A test tube, a lancet, a few labels. *Now* we would see. Now we would see what kind of man I am.

The testosterone testing kit had the potential to provide many answers. Despite what the 'experts' said, according to one corner of the Internet, male weakness, lethargy, fear, perhaps even snowflakedom itself, are down to a lack of testosterone. It could be the reason for my depressive tendencies, or on the other hand tell me what I'd always secretly suspected: that beneath this shell I was prime beefcake with a testosterone reading off the charts. With such revelations I would be free to reinvent myself as a biker or a cage fighter. I wouldn't *tell* anyone I had high testosterone, I'd just reveal it gradually, until one day Marian would turn to look at me only to find Jack Palance standing there, juggling kitchen knives and urinating into the dishwasher.

Following the instructions, I stabbed the lancet into my finger and squeezed drops of blood into the test tube. As the fourth and final drop of potent man blood dangled over the rim I started to feel faint. The kitchen tipped on its axis. On the verge of blacking out, I shook off the drop, then staggered deliriously up the swirling hallway like Catherine Deneuve in *Repulsion*. I grabbed a doorframe, then catapulted myself onto the sofa, where I rested my giant rock head on my seven-year-old son's shoulder.

I don't know much about Jack Palance, but I'm pretty sure if he lost four drops of blood he wouldn't have ended up imploring his child to 'fetch a biscuit before Daddy dies.' Not a good sign.

'Walking down the street of chance,' sang Iggy Pop in my ear. I turned the phone to watch the grainy video of him on stage at the Royal Albert Hall as I came out of the Tube, reluctant to fully accept the drab compromises of offline reality. The song ended and Iggy said, 'Everybody has a little voice inside them that says, "This path I'm on . . . does it have a heart or not?"'

I wasn't only worried about a heart, but about meat and muscle. Acquiring some.

In this I was somewhat behind the times. Over the last ten years the fitness industry in the UK has exploded, with the athletic legacy of the 2012 London Olympics, the arrival of advanced fitness technology and selfie-a-second social media display, with its attendant 'gymfluencers', all combining to make it worth an estimated £5 billion. Cycling clubs and Parkruns take over weekends, while more extreme challenges like Tough Mudder and ultra-marathons provide meaningful life events for thousands.

For the men in this country changing leisure time activities has led to changed bodies; pubs are disappearing, taking beer bellies with them. It could also show a desire to regain control over our physical states – to at least look like a man, until somebody figures out what the hell that means nowadays; protein shakes replacing little blue blankets as comforters.

My theory, however, is that there is more to it: that this urge towards training represents an emotional search as much as a physical one.

Drifting off Carnaby Street I walked into the Court Club, where I met Jason Fox. Foxy is one of a new breed of heavily muscled yet emotionally aware role models. People who are providing men with new kinds of messages.

It was early afternoon, and Jason was sipping mint tea in the bar, his clothes begging for mercy against the strain of his bulk. I sat opposite him like a pencil in front of a forest. Behind him was the stage where Jimi Hendrix had played an early gig with the Experience, when this venue was called the Bag o' Nails. Power and volume and performance: that's what Jimi was all about. Power and volume are what Foxy is known for too, but at the less flamboyant end of the spectrum.

Then again, nothing is ever quite what it seems. Not with Jimi, and not with Foxy. He knows all too well the gulf between outward appearance and internal disruption. An elite SBS (Special Boat Service) soldier with years spent barking orders at the toughest of the tough, one day he found he'd lost his drive and was diagnosed with PTSD, something he'd thought would never happen to him. He left active service and found himself cut adrift and in a dark spin. At the edge of a cliff one night, he found himself with a choice: rebuild his identity or face oblivion. Since he turned away from the brink he has achieved celebrity on the TV show *SAS: Who Dares Wins*, become a record-breaking Atlantic rower, and achieved various other feats to make most mortals look like slackers. Best of all, he has helped make the discussion of mental health acceptable even for the hardest of men.

What had worked for him, he told me, was going back to basics – finding himself a new tribe:

> When I was in the military, belonging to a group was just there as a by-product – you don't need to think about it. Then I left, and I was very, very down and alone, and I think it was because I wasn't part of a group. I missed that for a long period of time. Then I started to get back in touch with my mates. I did an Atlantic row on a team, where we were in a tribe for a time. Then I did *SAS: Who Dares Wins*, which periodically now supplies my tribal needs, and other bits like paddling the Yukon River, or going to the North Pole.

It doesn't sound much like back to basics, but it all sprang from a yearning for secure connections, which Foxy satisfied by reaching out to make friendships. His quest was underpinned by a discipline forged through physical exercise; a discipline over the self, over one's own worst instincts. 'Mentally it keeps me calm,' he said of his training regime. 'It's how I motivate myself. I'll get up before my alarm at five, which isn't nice, but I want that feeling after a session: the endorphins. A lot of it is to do with being conditioned in the military, where it's compulsory.' To him soldiering is akin to being a sportsman, in that it's a matter of commitment tied to an ambition to excel:

> When I went into military training at 16 it was the start of becoming a more professional, diligent individual. I wasn't like that

before, but I found something I loved. And it must be the same for boxers or athletes: they find something they like that gives them purpose. I thought, if I want to be good at something I need to concentrate, build up my skills and put time and effort into it. I wish I'd done that at school. If you've found your purpose, it instils discipline. You work your hardest to be good at it.

Foxy has covered a lot of ground in his life, but that mindset of discovering something you like and then putting everything into it has been the common thread. Purpose. That's what we all need, although it can be a cycle of losing it and gaining it; what no-one tells you is that purpose isn't permanent. In men's search for a solid identity, this can be earth-shattering: to grip life in your hands, only for it to slip through your fingers. 'After the military I'd lost my drive,' recalled Foxy.

It was difficult. I was floundering around for my purpose in life. It took a bit of time, but I think as a human you're allowed to have those lulls, because you're on a path that goes in different directions, and eventually you stumble across something else that you want to do well at.

To get through the difficult moments onto a new path you have to have support. 'No man is an island'? Just watch us try, hacking away sullenly at any shared ground. The worse you feel, the more you try to push yourself away into the fog of the open water. Conversely, one of the very positive aspects of male tribes, increasingly appreciated, is simply the arm around the shoulder. This consolatory role, now being taken on by men relaxed enough in their own masculinity to provide support for the duration, coming back to listen again and again, is where the future of male friendship lies.

Foxy told me about the gym he goes to, Manor, which is run by ex-boxers and cage fighters and has given him a genuine sense of belonging.

> Most of those lads are 15 years younger than me, but I love their company and we have a good laugh. It was another little thing which saved me from going mad. Not only do I get my physical kicks, I get to hang out with some lads who are like-minded. The Manor lads are fighters and can be bolshy and take the piss, but you can also sit down with pretty much all of them and say, 'I've had a bit of a 'mare.'

The fitness boom is sometimes characterized as a dumb 'spornosexual' trend (a media slur about high-street lads displaying pumped bodies modelled on sport and porn stars), when actually it is improving mental health by stimulating the release of feel-good chemicals and providing, in the course of an exercise routine, room to talk. Communities are created, connections made, and it's happening in all walks of life. Building-site workmates, office rivals, fathers and sons, grandfathers and granddaughters: all are finding expression as well as endorphin rushes. The old technique of sharing your troubles over twenty pints has not exactly disappeared, but an expanded arena of fitness spaces has become available for men to share regular time together, and with the bonus that you can actually remember the occasion afterwards. Jason from Sleaford Mods thought any remaining disdain for fitness revealed how rooted in the past people can be:

> I remember the guy from Franz Ferdinand tweeting, 'What musician goes to the gym?' And I just thought: you're quite an intelligent guy – why don't you do the maths? The time has gone

for rock 'n' roll excess. It's almost like how warfare changes: you don't bring a cannonball to a battle any more, brother.

Contrary to the macho image, even in the 'hardest' male settings there is more going on. During serious physical activity you need to be attuned to your emotions, too, in order to control them when confronted by a firefight, or a cage fight. Which is not the same thing as denying the emotion. 'In special forces you become emotionally aware because you have to,' reflected Foxy. 'I know when I'm scared, and I need to be aware of that to control it, otherwise I'll be a gibbering wreck. I'll go into it more – think: why am I scared? Even if it's just to realise I'm scared *because this is a scary situation!*'

Even the ultimate special forces warriors can access different masculinities. Since they fly around in helicopters with guns you might say their hardcore masculinity ticks so many boxes they are granted permission to do whatever they like. Nevertheless, now that some of their famous representatives are starting to reveal all the different ways of being a man, people are taking note. By giving men a positive direction that represents growth, not restriction, they are heralding a new era of aspiration. Foxy, who has been very open about his vulnerable moments, leaned in towards me:

Everyone says to me at the moment, 'It's all well and good *talking*, but what about being a bloke?' And I'm like, '*I'm* still a bloke.' I've got mates still in the Special Forces that are fucking hard, but we still check in with each other and talk about stuff. People are missing the point with the idea of having better 'soft' skills as a bloke: you're not removing anything, you're *adding* to it. It does my head in – you get people saying, 'Blokes don't do that.' Well, they've been saying that for years, but it's clearly not working, because people are topping themselves left, right and centre, so let's try and think outside the box . . .

The results of my testosterone test were in. I opened the email. 'The level of total testosterone in the sample you provided is 12.2 nmol/L (normal testosterone level: 7.6–31.4 nmol/L) This is a normal total testosterone level.'

I looked at the numbers a few times. *Not normal enough*, I decided. 12.2? Less than half the upper limit. This was intolerable.

Low T. The online 'manosphere' (the masturbatory male version of a knitting circle) bursts with memes and threads blaming any and all personal failings on a simple lack of the right chemicals:

Has your 'get up and go' got up and left?/
Low testosterone can cause low sex drive AND weight gain/
Heavy squatting and deadlifting SPIKES testosterone and human
   growth HORMONE by 530% for 48 hours/

A 'dark web' industry has sprung up to capitalize on such nonsense: get your testosterone, your crystal meth and your Uzi 9mm and that's you back on the right track of manhood. You *can* go down the NHS route but, as the illegal Viagra-derivative market showed, men would rather buy fake pills from gangsters than drop their trousers in front of a GP.

Dismissing both routes, I Googled how to improve testosterone levels without being prescribed injections. Exercise. Abstaining from sex. Abstaining from alcohol. We have two kids, so the middle one's no problem, and maybe the exercise could balance out the drink. I looked up Manor, and applied to join. Time to get in shape. No more physical weakness. For once in my daffodil life, it'd be good to feel physically big, like I could handle the trouble

I'd fantasized about. Not that I intended to seek trouble: I'd simply like to be ready for it in case it surprised me by the produce section at Waitrose.

Men are judged as physical specimens. Not in the same way as women, of whom society, as part of the need to subjugate an Other, reserves the right to be harshly judgemental. For men, physicality is another means of identifying a pecking order. While the support for men addressing their own fitness is admirable, it's not the whole story. Unless you have the classic 'ripped' figure you could find yourself outside any group support, and no less isolated. The Male Gaze exists for men as a pressure. Locker rooms are now parade grounds. The rise of penis fillers – Brotox, it's been called – and other enlargement techniques are fuelled by a desire not to improve sexual performance, but to avoid feeling ashamed when walking to a shower stall. Ab implants, steroid injections, waxing every bit of hair off your body . . . sure, if you're heterosexual there's an element of attracting the opposite sex, but impressing other men comes first. It is born out of that need to belong to a group, to be accepted, and validated as a man.

Dysfunction can result. Between 2010 and 2018 hospital admissions for adult men with eating disorders more than doubled, but even so, it's been estimated that less than 10 per cent of men living with an eating disorder seek professional help. Up to a million people in Britain use anabolic steroids for aesthetic reasons, not sport. There is a dark side to the broadly positive strides of the fitness boom, of new pressures bearing down. It doesn't take a paranoid technophobe to attribute these developments largely to the social media age, as the figures run in parallel to its rise to ubiquity: we are taking photos constantly, we are the subject of photos constantly, we are put on display for strangers to see constantly. We exist in a state of hyper-self-consciousness. Whose mental health can withstand the wild horses of identity performance pulling you apart? And, no, that's not a challenge to be met by a thousand Dwayne Johnson wannabes retorting, '*Bring it on, bubba . . .*'

Concrete walls. Thick air you could chew on. Sweat forcing itself out from inert pores. *Oh, my Christ.*

The main workout area of Manor turned out to be a converted car park. I was currently in a fight to the death with a large tyre. If I couldn't push it over it was going to fall backwards and kill me. Panicked, desperate for helpful advice, I glanced at a slogan stencilled on the wall beside me which read, '*Get the fuck on with it.*' Over the rim of the tyre I tried to spot my colleague Mark, hoping he was doing worse than me, but all I could see was Jason Fox walking my way. I gritted my teeth, heaved with the little strength I had left, and pushed the tyre past the tipping point till it fell. I followed suit in the other direction, flat on my back. Foxy's head appeared above me, upside down. He didn't say anything; he only laughed, with great, booming delight, and moved on.

My Manor membership hadn't been going well because I hadn't turned up to any sessions. Today, though, Mark and I had been invited to a workout Foxy was running as part of a brand launch. Based on no evidence at all I assumed I'd be able to cope, but it seemed every person on the planet was now a Terminator, and the level of exercise was so far beyond me I felt like a different species: some kind of sea slug flopping around on the floor. The others in my circuit training team, a breezy man and woman both built like Spartan warriors, helped me to my feet, seemingly only so I could watch both of them turn over the tyre as though it was a digestive biscuit. Nausea dropped through me. I grabbed my water bottle and approached a brass tap jutting out aggressively from the wall. As it spat water into my bottle I looked up and noticed another slogan: *'If you're looking for a mirror you're in the wrong fucking gym.'*

I turned and saw Mark yanking a thick rope up a long track. He was doing it with serious intent, his body locked in a solid frame, his teeth gritted in determination. A photographer had positioned himself to one side, capturing every moment of heroic struggle. Unbelievable. Mark exercised as much as I did – not at all – so how the shit was he managing that? I turned back to my team and stepped onto a treadmill to take my turn running at full pelt for thirty seconds. It sped up so fast that I had no choice but to match the pace, otherwise I'd fall and break my nose on the display. Even with my powers of self-delusion I knew I didn't look Instagrammable as I ran. I looked like a clothes horse trapped at the top of an escalator. Half a second before I had a heart attack so intense it'd defibrillate me back to life in the same instant, time was up. Wearing new liquorice legs I said, *I'm going to puke*, and followed the wall to the toilets, where I wailed impassioned ululations mourning the death of my dignity into the toilet bowl. Afterwards, I leaned my head against the hand dryer until I was confident the session would be over, then I went back out. Mark looked broken, but he was still standing for the warm-down.

I just puked, I told him.

Mark nodded as he stretched out his spine. 'I nearly did too, but on my way to the toilets, I thought: "No, I've got to help my team." So I went back.'

I thought, *That's the difference between me and you.*

On our way out we shook hands with Foxy, who laughed some more, and then in a moment of sudden affection I put my arm around Mark.

Shared struggle creates meaning between people. It is also about mutual admiration which is to do with physical transformation. Sweat is the amniotic fluid for our rebirth as He-Men. I came to understand this, not so much in the ashen aftermath of that first day, but in subsequent sessions as my panicked cardio-vascular system stopped rejecting my attempts to improve it. Hardcore exercise was about pain, going through pain together, and seeing the benefits of pain. It was about masochism, to a degree, and the chemical rush of exertion, but in terms of self-worth and group bonding, it was about authenticity. A man's desire to be the 'real deal'.

Even if being the 'real deal' is the ultimate MacGuffin – an undefined but highly motivating device – men have an almost spiritual yearning to attain that status. Building a ripped body is a very immediate way any man can show they are authentic. The biceps don't lie: they are real, you can touch them, and to achieve them you have to suffer. You can groom muscle, but you can't fake it (well, apart from ab implants, though with all due respect to the surgeons, the results usually look like six sausage rolls stuffed in a freezer bag). Heavy exercise is raw and real, it's manual labour on yourself.

That it may be only another kind of performance doesn't occur to most men. Indeed, suggesting this is often taken as an attack. This goes right to the heart of men's resistance to questioning masculinity: implying masculinity is something to be created as opposed to being a natural inevitability. It spoils the treasured quest to be the real deal, the striving for an authentic self. But such questioning is not an attack, nor a suggestion that such efforts are falsehoods or indeed don't matter – creating your own reality with a meaning that works for you is admirable; is all we godless types have in fact – rather it is a simple plea to acknowledge that it *is* created. Meeting classic masculine ideals with a hard-ass body is just one of many ways to express yourself, not necessarily *more* authentic than, say, becoming a willowy Goth. One's sense of being the real deal can come from a wide variety of personal values, and in the area of physicality, it could come from making peace with however your body is, even if it doesn't meet a certain societal standard.

I was some way off realising this at that time.

For me, as I found myself grunting with effort and confusion over free weights, I began to enjoy the sense of a growing control over my body. Personally, it wasn't about getting stacked – mind you, looking less like a stack of pancakes was nice – I simply wanted confidence in my physicality, when my body has always been something I'm ashamed of.

Most male role models are defined by the body, not the mind. Our ideals are physical ideals. Actors and sportsmen with bodies like gods. Again, it is that association with authenticity: popular idols for men need to 'walk the walk', and shed blood, sweat and tears. A premium is put on very physical, active forms of leadership. Nothing wrong with that, except to say that body and mind should be valued together.

With boys there is shame attached to improving your mind in a way that there never is when it comes to the body: if you're clever, you either deny it or hide it, and, as soon as you can, ruin it all with booze. Those that display it proudly, well . . . best of luck out in the playground. It's tragic, awful, absurd but true, that intellect is cause for many a young man to be bullied. The emphasis for young lads is all on the body: whoever is strongest, fittest, sportiest – these are the ones who rule a school. Humour, manipulation and wisecracks are of course all valued expressions of intelligence, but the notion of sitting down to study hard has mostly been seen as a bit perverted. The game is to *not* try, to not care. Boys are falling behind girls at every level of education, and that is partly because of the peer culture of boys, and parental emphasis on more physical presentations of male achievement. That girls forge ahead in education only to be confronted by a wage gap in employment is a sickener which appears to support the conclusion that men aren't valued for their brains but for, well, just being men.

In taking on such injustices, feminist messaging has filtered down to young girls, culturally and socially, putting new value on empowerment. Encouragement to reach beyond society's gender expectations appears to be reaching girls, but not boys. Instead, boys are rarely educated on evaluating or transcending any gender confines. As the 'standard' humans, the ruling males, boys are assumed to have things their own way; why bother intervening? But as we've seen with mental health, if boys are left to their own devices – 'Oh, they're fine' – it can be severely detrimental. What's more, the fight for equality can't only be communicated to the girls – if you want change, the boys need to understand the issue too.

Part of this is about supporting boys in their exploration of a variety of masculinities. The positive messaging which does reach boys is generally around sport: the language of 'resilience', 'team spirit' and 'determination' – all valuable qualities, and indeed sport can build confidence and a sense of self for anyone, regardless of background or intelligence level or ability. The only problem is that positive affirmations in other areas of life are thin on the ground.

You never hear boys being told they 'smashed it at kindness today'. Or 'knocked the algebra out of the park'.

The popular role models we point boys towards are generally the sporting types too: the figures on TV, on magazine covers and in advertising campaigns, identified as swaggering machines, with no need for brains and above emotions. This is the kind of propaganda which creates dominant male fictions. Actually, top sportsmen achieve their success because they are trained not just physically but intellectually and, most importantly, emotionally. We are only sold half the story about such people, shown the end result but not the process. The best boxers, for example, spend inordinate amounts of time on their minds – look at Muhammad Ali, whose genius came in outwitting opponents – yet it's very rare for them to be exhibited as anything other than big hard bastards.

This is not to decry sport's position in male aspiration; in fact, it is to celebrate the opportunity it has afforded in the last few years to expand the parameters of masculinity. Which brings us back to the shape-shifting effects of social media age: sportsmen have been able to shine a light on their lived realities, the role of friends and family in their training, to reveal the complexities of being a man. This is one of the most promising things to happen to men in the modern age. It's no accident that the greatest taboo-busters in male mental health are sports stars, because they are both the most visible role models and assumed to have the least going on in their heads, which is far from the truth.

The mentality of Hull boxer Luke Campbell MBE, an Olympic gold medal winner, has to be drum-tight. He was in London to get treatment on a bicep when I met him. He was sitting in

Pret A Manger, quietly eating porridge while the workers in Hammersmith queued for buckets of coffee, and the first thing I noticed about him were his wide grey eyes, which seemed to exude a sharp light as he evaluated his surroundings. I wanted to speak to him about the mind of a boxer; why you can be in the shape of your life but still lose if your head's not right.

Single-mindedness was his superpower, he told me, but it is a constant battle with yourself:

> With the pressure I put on myself to succeed, to perform, to win, the negatives can come flooding in: 'Am I fit enough?', 'Hope I don't get knocked out', 'What if I go down?' In the Olympics I developed my own mental preparation: I wouldn't let myself think about what's going to happen in the fight ahead. It gets my nerves going. I don't need the adrenaline before; I just need to concentrate on the present. A lot of athletes at the Olympics folded with the pressure, but I developed the 'fuck it' attitude. *I don't care.* That put me in a place where I was all right. Obviously I *did* care, and I wanted to win *so* much, but I thought 'Fuck it, if I give it 100 per cent I'm not bothered, I can live with myself.'

Luke spoke about what goes through his mind in the ring, and why you have to attune to your emotions in order to stay in control:

> You can't be angry – you'll get knocked out. If you lose your calmness, you lose your concentration, make mistakes and get hit. You don't want to be thinking too much in the ring: it's a reaction game. If he throws a jab you have to react by slipping it, then hitting at the same time. Your body will react the way it's been trained to do.

This is the 'flow state' often referred to in sport psychology. When mind and body are together, allowing clarity beyond thought.

It's the feeling every sportsman chases – that every person chases, in fact: achieving such complete concentration in what you are doing that you forget any notion of the self and act without thinking about it, in almost a dream state. Despite the chaos of masculinity today, the ultimate personal goal may well be the same as it's ever been: finding something that allows you to rise above any human concerns to touch godliness 'in the zone'.

'I've got good focus,' Luke said. 'You hear everybody say to kids, "Concentrate!" But no-one ever *teaches* them how to concentrate. I do drills with my youngest son – ladder fitness drills, or even just counting out a big bag of shrapnel – to get his mind focused.' Even such small moments of concentration can open up an area of bliss that, when the modern world bombards you with its demands from an alarmingly young age, is very desirable.

In a pressurized world of instant, visible achievement people rush for short cuts. But excellence doesn't work like that. Quick fixes can only lead to disillusionment and envy. How other people have attained their success is all over social media, but if you want it too, you have to reach for it as hard as they did. Reaching suggests improvement. Improvement requires determination. To not simply fantasize, but to commit to the relentless, repetitive work to get there, and understand it as a process of learning. This allows people like Luke to remain bulletproof. He was fresh out of his fight with Vasyl Lomachenko, one of the greatest fighters ever. Against many predictions Luke held his own, took it the distance and gave Lomachenko some real problems. But what happened in the aftermath?

Everybody came up to me and said, 'Well done – you must be so proud!' And I was like, 'I lost . . . I'm not proud.' I have my own goals, and if I don't hit them I need to go back and practise. I need

125

to be getting better. After every fight, I go back to basics: a jab, foot position, go right back. People get caught up in so much, when you need to simplify. With everything in life it's always good to remind yourself: go back to basics.

That getting-back-to-basics again. Seeking to improve. Athlete methodology – or Foxy's Special Forces mindset if you prefer – can be applied to your own life, including in your darkest moments when you're spinning away from the light. Before he left, I asked Luke for his favourite bits of advice: 'The SAS – and *Only Fools and Horses* – one: "He who dares, wins". Oh, and: "Fuck it."'

A 'Fuck It' attitude may be a great thread of male achievement. While the clichés that men are 'simple creatures' or 'don't listen' are irritating, they may reflect of a tendency in men to be very single-minded in their pursuits to the detriment of everything else. At least, that's my new excuse. But in its most positive aspect, of being driven, concentrating on your own endeavour, and *not worrying about the consequences*, it is surely what brings together footballers, artists, scientists, anyone in that moment in their lives when they really go for it.

Fuck it.

Often it can be disastrous, too. When you're faced with a Ukrainian granite-man about to punch you in the face it's not a bad Zen strategy, but when you're on a charity walk with no training, it's stupid. The same talent for excluding all else in the pursuit of a dream, denying doubt, can also lead down lonely paths of delusion. Reality can bite hard. The trick may just be to understand this tendency and channel it, without removing the impulse altogether. And not embarking on your challenges alone: keep the support around you. If masculinity is relational then transformations of masculinity have to be too: we're all in it together.

Early evening in the grotty basement of an expensive craft beer pub. Luke was seated by me, along with fellow boxer Dave Allen and ex-rugby pro Kearnan Myall. I wrapped up the panel chat we'd had about mental health and passed the mic to Freddie Flintoff, who had come to the stage. I sat back on my stool behind him. Too close behind him. The way Freddie planted himself meant if he took even half a step backwards he'd sit on my knee and we'd have a ventriloquist act. As he began speaking, I deftly slipped through his armpit and into the shadows.

Flintoff has the enviable ease of a public figure used to having people listen. He eyed up the room and began:

> Every time on a cricket field I walked about there as if I owned the joint – but at no point did I ever feel like that . . .
>
> When I was playing, I thought the idea of telling someone about that would've been weakness. My view on mental strength is very different these days. It is the ability to talk, to tell people how you feel, and probably more importantly to tell the people around you. The relationships I have with my friends now are very different . . .
>
> If you take nothing else from this event, just think about how you talk to people. Think about your relationship with your family, with your friends. What do you talk about? Do you know your mates really? Do you know what they're going through? And if not, why not try to find out?

This kind of talk from national sporting heroes is undoubtedly new. On the eve of the last World Cup a number of England players talked about mental health struggles, fully supported by their manager Gareth Southgate; twenty, even five, years ago this would have been unthinkable. But Flintoff has headed a breakthrough in how sporting figures are perceived, backed by campaigns from charities like CALM and Heads Together which sporting authorities are bringing into stadiums. They reveal the frailties of our idols, and how 'normal' men may view their own frailties. Once again, the route to publicly expanding masculinity into an emotional dimension has been mental health, and the mental health of our previously impregnable athletic warriors.

Kearnan Myall is massive: 6 foot 7, a former Wasps player who hit the papers for breaking ranks by revealing his struggles with depression. We were talking at another event, a staff session on mental health at a media agency. Kearnan told us about being an elite athlete and in the system since he was nine. 'It's a great feeling to push yourself to the limit and to see other people put their bodies on the line for you – it inspires you to do the same. And it means a team can reach bigger heights than its individual members.' His career rose to international level, but then a personal relationship ended and he started experiencing depression. Off the pitch, a switch had been flipped, and he launched into self-destructive partying; a common but not often talked about sign of depression that's a consequence of not caring for yourself, and actually a form of self-harm.

On the pitch, though, things were fine: 'I could never understand why I played the best rugby of my career while I was suicidal.' Training was more difficult. Something was badly wrong, but he hid it.

I couldn't let the coaches think I was struggling, otherwise I wouldn't be picked. Before going into training I'd park at the far end of the car park, stay in the car, and cry it all out there, so I

128

wouldn't cry in front of the others. Then I'd avoid eye contact. Get through it.

It all came to a head when he tested positive for cocaine after a random drugs test – retrospectively he thinks that was what saved him. He was sent off to a psychiatrist, who diagnosed him with depression, and set him on a path to recovery. 'When it came to mental health issues I thought I was on my own, I was the only crazy one. It was only when I went to get help I was told it was perfectly common, especially because of the circumstances.'

Kearnan is currently studying for a PhD on mental health support for athletes. For it clearly isn't there now. Jonny Benjamin, whom we met earlier, told me he went to see a top Premier League club about giving a talk, but was told by the club psychologist he wouldn't be able to mention suicide – kind of tricky when you're Jonny. 'I said to the psychologist, "I don't understand – these are grown men and they need to hear it." And he said, "We have to wrap them up in cotton wool. Imagine if these players are open about their problems: they'd get so much abuse on a Saturday." Organizational fear at the top level is holding back support for players and, as a consequence, for anyone who looks up to them as role models. The priority is protecting their players in the short term, thereby protecting the club's investments.

I asked Kearnan to enlarge on why he could still perform on the pitch despite all his troubles off it, and his response chimed with what Luke had to say about the 'flow state'.

Once you run out on the pitch and the whistle goes, all anxiety disappears. It's like a calm sea in your mind. Even though it's hectic and you're charging about, smashing into people, shouting and swearing, in your mind you're calm and comfortable. It's the best feeling in the world.

Afterwards, Kearnan and I went for a walk in the City during the lunchtime rush hour. Thanks to his sheer size we managed to carve out a bit of room in a coffee shop to talk. I was after his take on why there has been such an explosion of extreme physical exercise in recent years, and whether it's a response to the technological advancements of the modern world. He nodded.

The lives we are living now are so far removed from what we're evolved to do. The rate technology has advanced over last 20 years has completely transformed our lives. Evolution is not even close to catching up. A lot of the anxieties we face are because our brains focus on the threats around us. When we were hunter-gatherers, and even when we were more advanced and living in societies, in order to stay alive people whose brains focused on threats were more likely to thrive. In day-to-day life now generally we're extremely safe, yet our brains are still focusing on the threats. We see danger in things that aren't actually a risk to our health: having a bad meeting with a manager, a public speech, someone looking at you funny on the street. Perhaps there's a link to why people want to do aggressive sport – because it helps deal with some of those anxieties.

Lord knows I needed some release from my anxieties. Why does aggressive sport have to be the answer, though? And not something at which I am more adept: cupcake eating? Moaning?

I was back at Manor, shirking out of a session again, but with good reason: it's hard to deadlift when your arms are overcooked linguini.

'C'mon, Martin – get into it, for fuck's sake!' Chris Baugh was waving from the door, giving me his usual form of encouragement. He's the co-founder of Manor, and an ex-boxing pro. Before I showered I grabbed him for a chat in his office along with another member who everyone seems to call 'the Magic Marine'. By now, as I asked them about the mindset the gym can foster, I was revelling in my recurrent role as the least hard man in the room.

Chris said they'd deliberately set up Manor to be a place with no macho nonsense, which he said was common to proper fighting gyms:

> I've been kickboxing in spit and sawdust gyms since I was 15 – I switched to boxing at 18. There's something about fighting environments that may be intimidating, because there's no tolerance for excuses, but actually, because everyone's like-minded, there's a lot of warmth and community. There's nothing to be gained from shouting about your toughness. At Manor, we expect you to walk in without a sense of entitlement, and not swaggering around trying to boss people about. This is a community, and you have to be with our values, which are humility, kindness, openness and positivity.

There's something about fitness activity which creates tribes of a different nature from your typical old-school pub gang. Hard physical graft is about self-improvement, which requires mutual encouragement, which in turn encourages the sharing of thoughts, problems and anxieties. Exactly what men need. Part of this was also about not being a purely male environment, Chris said: membership is 60–40 men to women. And though we are concentrating on the male experience, what is absolutely central to the fitness boom is that it is creating shared experiences for all genders, which of course creates a diverse environment in which men's masculinities are likely to flourish.

Chris saw the marketing messages spread to men and women in the modern age as one of the reasons why their communication is working.

> The fitness industry sells to people using shame and guilt: 'You shouldn't look how you look. Here's a picture of someone who you're nothing like: you should look like them.' It makes you in awe of it, but then you buy the product or service, find you don't know how to do it properly, then start to feel even shittier about yourself. Don't look at [extreme athlete] Ross Edgley now: look at what he did 10 or 20 years ago to build up to it.

The other major aspect of the new appetite for extreme fitness is connected with the blinkers-on grind of modern working life for a great many men. Even if you've drifted up the ladder by the usual routes, you can discover it isn't what you thought: that the rewards on the outside have done nothing for your inside. 'The "game" is hollow,' said Chris.

> Everyone that I know who has succeeded at the game has turned around at some point and gone, 'Do you know what? I've got it all, but what the fuck have I done with my life? I don't think I've worked for it or asked any hard questions of myself. This is where I've ended up. I've got the girl, got the house, got the car, got the kid, got the dog – now fucking what?'

The way Chris saw it, if comfort dampens down ambition and spirit, then you have to regularly take the step the other way.

> We have to practise discomfort. Our head coach has had us doing cold showers every day this month. Thirty seconds, then a minute,

then up to two minutes by the end of the month. It's about under-standing that the way you feel is only half the picture. Athletes know that, fighters know that, soldiers know that – because they all have to go through things that they don't want to. Discomfort is about discipline.

At this point the Magic Marine spoke up, about how this kind of discipline can help with a self-destructive streak, as it's helped him with his drinking.

We're geared to be working and reacting. When you're living a comfortable, calm life there's nothing to react to. We're not supposed to be like that, so we throw a bag of spanners in the works and react to it. We've got all these mechanisms inside us that have evolved to react to stimulus, so we don't really want a calm life.

I thought of this as both disturbing and right on the money. Men's self-destructive streaks can be linked to boredom, ennui, along with an impulse to see what happens if . . . People want challenge in their lives, and if it's not happening elsewhere a lot of destruc-tion, I'd argue, comes from needing to create it in their personal lives. If it takes cold showers and hitting a tyre with a hammer to supply the daily challenges, so much the better. Potentially, the rush to fitness and adventure can create fulfilment in a way that working lives never could. It speaks to a need not to settle for the drift of life, but to do something more meaningful. In this respect it is truly existential: a search for a reality beyond the one you have been presented with. And to act on it, as so many are doing, is to signify a triumph over society, bosses, parents and gender. It is an escape from the prison of ourselves.

'Make sure you come to my boxing session on Friday,' Chris said to me on the way out. 'I'm going to see you there this week, right?'

He always says this to me, and I said, *I'll be there*, like I always do. But I won't be.

The first time I'd gone to book a boxing session I'd seen that you have to bind your hands with tape, and that if you haven't done it before a trainer would help you. Which counted me out.

My left hand is deformed.

I have three fingers instead of five. I was born this way and have spent a lifetime hiding it.

Bodies are the source of men's perceived as well as actual power. An emphasis on the performance of the male body from a very young age makes it arguably the first route to glory or failure. The pressures of society hit you young – at school, from family and friends, your environment, your class, colour or sexuality – and can leave people with a lot of psychological scars. But as adults, we can now seek solutions by circling back to training, sport and adventuring. It is possible.

However, some scarring lasts a lifetime, and needs further care.

My left hand is like some malevolent force existing beyond my vision, like a ghost more sensed than seen. I have become so used to never acknowledging it that for me it almost doesn't exist, or only in the manner that memories exist, or fear. Even though my hand is a part of the bone and flesh of my body, the way I came to deal with it was by pretending nothing was amiss. Clever me – that solved it! If a kid came up to me in the playground to ask me if the rumours were true that I had 'a three-fingered hand' I'd simply deny it. Keep it in my pocket and say, 'Bollocks.' In all the years since this strategy hasn't really changed. I'll still hide it away out of habit to such an extent that on the rare occasions when somebody does spot it, it's almost more shocking for me than for them: *Jesus! When did that happen?*

The reason that it is a malevolent force, not a benign one, is simply that its existence in my mind, separated from reality as I'd decided reality should be, gave it immense power over me. It wasn't mere twisted flesh: it was mythic. What could have been an insignificant barrier to a normal life became instead something too terrible to bear because I chose to hide it. Nobody forced me to, not even the mean kids or grown-up arseholes along the way: it was my choice. And, well, it messed me up. Not to a place beyond hope, but enough to keep me in that silent, depressed state, a dysfunctional unhappiness, for way too many years, which even now I find hard to shake. Relationships, family and friends were lost to the void at the end of my sleeve. I think I never came close to finding who I was because I was too busy hiding myself away.

It was nobody's fault but mine. Still, I have come to consider that my actions were not purely independent – I am not, I think, completely insane – but rather bound up in my environment and, since I was male, masculinity.

I was ashamed of my hand. That shame was the core impulse to hiding the thing. And shame can only exist under the gaze, or prospective gaze, of other people. Whereupon, you assume, you will be judged against the standard you see elsewhere. All those beautiful hands! I used to look at other people's fingers playing guitar, or forming bridges on pool tables, or filling up a glove in its entirety, or linking hands with a girl – fascinated. I didn't feel resentment; only a longing to be able to do the same. That I had one 'good' hand, and could probably have managed to play guitar, or even linked hands with a girl using my 'bad' hand, was, in my distorted reality, lost on me. These days I look at the little hands of my son and my daughter enraptured: such a great abundance of fingers! It's strange, but it's like their fingers are mine, too, and I can feel what they feel. I *love* this. I love that having their full quota of digits is at least one less thing to worry about in a world of worries.

The shame, though: the shame was undeniably linked to not feeling like a complete person, not like the other boys. Whenever my hand was referenced during my primary school years, it seemed as though no-one really cared about it one way or the other, so I didn't care either. When puberty hit, however, as self-consciousness dug its claws in and I became aware of my developing body and mind, and where I might fit in the world . . . then everything fell apart. I felt there was no hope for me: that I was hideous, abject, cursed in some way. I hated my hand, and hated myself, so the only way to carry on was to pretend it didn't exist. And if I could blend in with the other boys and later, among other men, conform to whatever was necessary to pass for Normal, then I needn't be a freak. So long as I kept the damn thing out of sight.

Well, you learn how to do that easily enough: keep the bad hand in the pocket wherever possible, carry only one pint at a time from the bar, avoid pool, don't wear gloves in winter to avoid Floppy Finger Syndrome, and make use of folded arms, coats, tables, whatever you can, to hide it. Life was at a remove; chatting in the pub while at the same time making sure no-one was looking down at it. If eyes did settle on you, then adjust, shift position, tuck it away and keep smiling.

The quieter I was, I found, the less people looked, and so tightly did this wrap itself around my psyche that most of the time I was as close to invisible as you could get.

The feeling I had was of being Other. Despite taking the straight white male road to career respectability, I felt absolutely different. It was this, I suppose, that made me see masculinity in a different light: something to be at first consciously sought, then as I grew in experience and saw its limitations and lies, rejected. I saw how men operated on the basis of Us versus Them, of Normal versus Other, of standard humans and those who are less than human. And there came a point when I didn't want to be a part of that, because I saw – knew – the damage it can cause. Worse, I realised I had colluded in it, and betrayed my Other status. I had sold it out, fearing to lose what being disguised as Normal granted me. This is hard to admit. A world of division and hate depends on such cowardice.

Countless men undoubtedly feel themselves in some way different to what we're supposed to be. But can we stop hiding it and then take it all the way? Can we *celebrate* the Other aspects of ourselves? And then, critically, help those who are considered Other through common prejudice become part of a new, kaleidoscopic Normal?

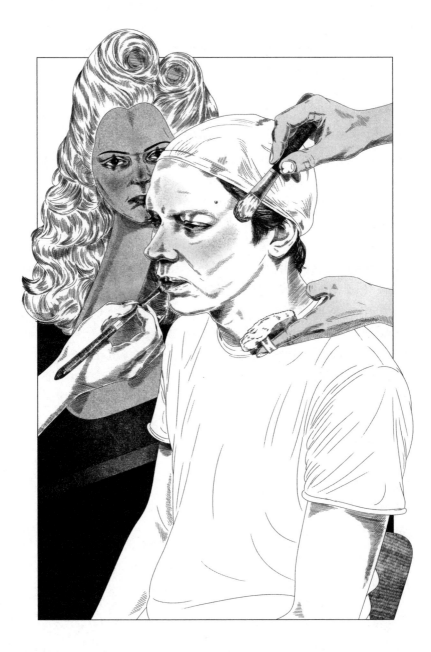

5

You Are Straight

Sexuality, Women and the Other

Alien-queen eyes stared into mine. Cheddar Gorgeous was before me. Her eyes were covered with jet-black lenses, the same colour as her lips, which were pursed in concentration. The foundation was getting plastered on my face thick and fast now. The dome of her perfectly shaven and whitened head reflected the light as she worked. I was banned from looking in the mirror until the make-up was finished, which was fine with me, because I was afraid to. I was way out of my cishet fuckboy element, crawling out of my silent shell into the flamboyant landscape of camp. My hands were tucked firmly under my thighs.

'The thing about being gay is that a lot of the time it's something you have to hide away, right?' said Cheddar, in her thick Mancunian accent.

But drag is about making yourself visibly different. And it means you become a spectacle, which brings people together to communicate. It's why drag has played such a role in articulating the gay rights movement, because you need people to lead the charge in drawing attention to issues.

Lipstick was applied next. Bar the odd Halloween party I hadn't worn any since my early twenties, and the glorious glam rock week when I ditched my nerves, hit the lippie and eyeliner and rocked it like Iggy Pop in the farthest corner of the darkest pub in town. I felt much more compromised now, with years of calcified adult manliness built up; besides, this wasn't mere flirtation with glamour but a commitment, a transformation beyond my normal confines. The more make-up went on, the more exposed I felt.

Cheddar and her entire 'drag family' were giving journalists a taste of their world to promote a TV show called *Drag SOS*, which helped people climb out of personal holes with a sequined rope ladder. The participants tended to be low-confidence souls in need of love and care, or straight dads who connected with their gay offspring by taking part in a drag show. It was a window into a world of changing perceptions. As she glued butterflies to my temples Cheddar told me about a 'very masculine' rugby player from Wales who went through the experience for his children: 'He wanted them to grow up thinking you can be many different ways in the world. I thought that was fantastic.'

Next, a wire headpiece Cheddar had crafted at home was fixed onto me. It was covered in fruit, flowers and more butterflies. As she pressed it into my temples she asked me which part of the whole experience was making me uncomfortable. And I'd thought I was hiding it so well. *The exposure*, I told her, *on a personal level. And I suppose as a straight man you're taught from a young age not to dress anything like this. You're supposed to be natural, no frills.* 'So why did you want to try drag?' *To push against the boundaries of what we are taught as men. And I need more Instagram followers.*

As I sat there I recalled the gay friends I had become close to over the years, particularly those I'd worked and lived with in my early twenties. My attraction to them could well have been sexual, but I think it was mostly about their sense of identity. While I floundered for a sense of who I was, the process of coming to terms with their sexuality, and coming out to friends and family, had, it appeared, given them a confidence about who they were. They had a strength of character, no doubt developed through some tough times, that was missing in my straight friends. Secretly I empathized with what they had been through, knowing a little of the feeling of difference they felt. Not that I opened up to them, but I hoped to acquire some of their strength – that is, without revealing my own little secret, obviously.

With all this in mind, I confessed to Cheddar that I was also worried I didn't have it in me to camp it up properly for the role.

'I don't think that's right, though,' she objected. 'Drag that tries too hard can be bad drag. So many people go into it thinking you should have a formulated caricature, and I don't think that's what drag's about. It's about allowing you to feel comfortable to be whoever you feel like being. It's about expression.'

Cheddar stepped to one side to allow Tete Bang to take over. Tete is a woman in drag – a lesser-known type of drag queen, but not a rarity – and she told me how it provided her with a way to explore her personality, which while she'd been growing up hadn't been deemed very feminine: she wasn't the way 'girls' should be.

> I'm from a rural, working-class town in the Lake District, and came out as gay when I was 15. It was really shit. I suffered from mental health problems, and my last-ditch attempt at survival was to move to London. I worked in a chip shop and saved up to move down here. I was always into costumes, and I basically used to make

outfits and go to the [iconic gay venue] Black Cap in Camden by myself. Before I knew it I was part of a community. I didn't realise that's what I was looking for all that time. I'd always been told that I'm a bit much, too loud, too annoying – all those things a woman isn't supposed to be. I think I wasn't loud and annoying: I was just a drag queen.

While this story of finding a new identity beyond the one you were supposed to have, along with a new community to validate it, was inspiring, it had taken plenty of suffering to get there. Simply having a 'different' sexuality, or being 'different' from gender expectations, makes life tough for you. 'Different' still meaning: a divergence from the Default Male.

My make-up was finished. I was helped into a corset which made me stand up straight for the first time in decades. Over the top Cheddar draped a kimono. I had never worn a kimono before. They don't hide much, do they?

'OK, are you ready to have a look in the mirror?"

I think so.

I turned for the moment of truth. As the kimono spun around my frame, I had the uncanny sensation of not recognizing myself in a mirror.

Martin Robinson was different. Martin Robinson was ... beautiful.

More than that, actually. I wasn't merely gorgeous, I was a work of art. Well, usually I look like something in a Francis Bacon painting, but at that moment I was a background figure from Botticelli, only with hairy arms and leg spots.

The drag-over was not yet complete, though: I also had to climb into 6-inch heels. Up I went onto them, arms outstretched, as Cheddar bound my feet into place. *Lord, why have you forsaken me?* At 6 foot 2 already, an extra 6 inches of height caused the fruit on my head to freeze in the grille of the air-conditioning unit. I was beckoned forward, but immediately collapsed to the ground like an early flying machine. If ever a man wants evidence of the psycho-sexual sadism society subjects women to, put him in a pair of heels. It's like having to go about your daily business with each foot in a live goose.

I was taken down a flight of stairs and across a studio, whimpering in the panic of the newly birthed, to have my photo taken. I couldn't go more than one step without turning my ankle and toppling. Only by having Cheddar and Tete hold me on either side to place me in different positions could I get through the shoot. 'Come on, blow some kisses,' said the photographer. *I am in fear of my life, sir,* I hissed between mwahs.

Reprieved at last, I was propped up against a wall while the other dragged-up journalists were photographed. Left alone in my silent stillness I was more a plinth than a person. It was strange of me to resort to my usual invisibility technique when I was, you know, IN FULL DRAG. I started to feel down. Being a living spectacle is at the other end of the spectrum from where I like to be, but it wasn't simply that: it was disappointment that I wasn't rising to the occasion. Despite what Cheddar had told me, I'd imagined my physical transformation would unleash a hilarious, outgoing, wildly camp side: a touch of Wildean wit, a dash of Bowie-esque swagger – but it didn't. It made me shrink. What was wrong with me? If you gave me the keys to a chocolate factory I'd start producing cardboard.

Cheddar helped me down off the heels and into a chair for a cup of tea. Butterflies dropped off my face as I swallowed my failure and asked her why drag was proving so popular on TV, with their

143

show and others like *RuPaul's Drag Race.* 'Our society is attracted to the visual,' she said.

> Maybe because of the role in social media in forming our friend-ships and the way we communicate. We're becoming more nuanced in the way we express our identity visually, so it makes sense that drag queens are having a moment right now. And why should that be something only gay men can benefit from?

But are heterosexual men anywhere near ready to?

When it comes to culture there is a glory in Outsiderdom. A defiance of mainstream sensibilities that you see in almost all great art. And I saw it in this drag family, as they gathered at the Formica table to eat biscuits under the cold strip lights: a fresco of exploding lampoonery by self-imagined Pop Art creatures busy undercutting it all with putdowns delivered in the same bone-dry drawl. Searching for the extraordinary far from what was expected of them, carrying a degree of pathos as a nod to their exclusion, and darting out the kind of barbed wit that comes from knowing the truth about a cowardly world. Their quest is for brave new modes of living where the rest of us fear to tread. Gay culture's influence on art, fashion, music, humour, is incalculable – it would be absurd to try and list it. Collective British identity springs directly from it.

So why is the fight for rights and representation for LGBTQ+ communities still so hard-fought? We have reaped the rewards of this outsider culture, yet they continually have to come from a position of being unacceptable as people.

One reason, it seems to me, is that straight men, insulated by their neutral centre of privilege, are doing nowhere near enough to support communities who are different from them; who have 'failed' in this sense to be Normal. It has been up to the Other to protest, while the Default Male affects to listen . . . and so the gears of equality grind interminably slowly.

For any real change to occur the world has to end. The world as you know it, that is: the one you would normally experience when you leave the house and which you barely even register as you suck on your frappuccino. It means the end of your identity, your life-style, your security. Change is frightening. Real change, that is, not a new haircut or an Instagram post in support of the day's most digestible political issue; real change which alters lives.

Equality for all, with the freedom that follows, is surely the unifying goal we can all agree on, the thing to protect against extremists. It is not a new idea; it's bound up in constitutions, manifestos, laws, to an extent – so why haven't we achieved it? Equality in real terms, that is: social terms, employment terms, cultural involvement. For instance, in the UK the gender pay gap has been calculated to cost women £140 billion a year in pay.

It begs the question: do people actually want equality?

And by 'people' I mean men.

Do we actually want change?

Which brings us to the idea of self-analysis for men. A hard look at oneself. 'What do I really stand for?'

The danger right now – a time of flux, one of those historical periods when rapid technological development calls politics, society, nations, personal identities, all into question – is that the opportunity to seize equality will be lost. The prize of human freedom for everyone will slip away because it won't have been fought for. Not in a critical area, the centre ground, among those who have the power: the Default Males, who had the means to make real change happen but didn't.

The end of your world. A lot of men shudder at the thought, shudder at the patriarchy coming under attack, shudder at the very term 'patriarchy': *There's no such thing . . . What a load of nonsense.'* I get it: I've been guilty of that – selling out my own difference to stay comfortable. I'm one of a mass of people just trying to get along as best I can. It's hard to break out from your own narrow concerns. And yet the opportunity is there for a life better than the one we know, for everyone.

Masculinity is not pathological, but it can be neurotic. The process of societal Other-ing has its roots in this aspect of masculinity. In a country like the UK, with a historically dominant white heterosexual male population, it is straightforward: anyone who is non-heterosexual, non-male, non-white is Other. This neurosis lumps everyone in together: women, LGBTQ+ communities, Black people, Asian people, disabled people . . . all of whom are simply, well, *wrong* – for not being the standard human. It comes from a narrowed perspective, which for men can be learned from a very young age. As we've seen, part of the way masculinity works is to restrict male identity to old nostalgic forms which are safe, easy to understand and easy to police. Within this there is room to shift, sure, room to stand apart, more than meets the eye, but it's difficult to escape it: it's drummed into us very early on to identify what's different and reject it, in order to firm up our own identities. It is deep in the male psyche – but not deep enough that it should be left alone.

The idea of Othering has its origins in the relation of man to woman. Beginning with the Creation story of Adam and Eve. A woman was pulled out of the side of the *original* human, who then proceeded, after five minutes of showing off her body in the garden, to get chatting to some snake and then ruin everything.

Untrustworthy, lowly women – sinners from the start! *It's enough to make a man forever suspicious of anyone who looks different* . . .

Using opposition to form an identity is deep-rooted – you see it in small children who seek to define who they are by rejecting what they are not. Sample conversation with my daughter: 'That's for babies . . . that's a boy toothbrush . . . that's for girls with yellow hair . . . no, Daddy, just *no*.' Yet you'd expect there to come a time when it matures. But the male neurosis of Other-ing prevents this. For men very concerned with demonstrating their manliness – the 'correct' way of behaving – you have to be seen to reject the Other in all forms. If you're not careful, your whole life becomes a performance of Being A Man, restricting the ability to live as a fully-rounded person,and restricting the freedoms of fellow humans.

The call for equality will keep echoing around without being translated into reality because it appears *men don't really want it*. Certainly not those with the power to do something about it but who are too afraid of losing that power. Often the support of equality can amount to a feint. 'Smash the patriarchy!' – *but not today, thanks*. 'Appoint more black people!' – *but only a couple, for the quota*. 'Support gay pride!' – *but no, son, you can't go to the parade*.

This male neurosis is a neurosis of power. It comes from looking over your shoulder. Appeasing dissent while keeping control.

But how can we change this? By surrendering. ('*Say, what?*') Surrendering what we have learned about the way a man should be in the world, and sticking out a hand for those in need.

If we want to explore more masculinities then letting go is a good place to begin. Happiness can be sought not from power but from co-operation and inclusion. Otherwise the neurosis of power is all that concerns us. And I think this preoccupies men to such a degree – the public show of being a man and fighting for control – that it is the major cause of dysfunction. Surrendering control, then, is the route to more freedom for all, including freeing men from themselves. Sharing that power. That it requires men bold enough to dismantle the structures that favour them is obvious. And today it's what we lack.

I was at a large employer's lunchtime session, talking about why men should be more open while telling them nothing about what was really bothering me. As ever at such masculinity events encouraging men to talk, the audience was 95 per cent women. It made me wish I was truly opening up, so I could be righteously indignant.

On I went – one hand behind my back – talking generally about depression, ad-libbing it, by which I mean waffling, until I tailed off and sat down next to the other men on stage, who had talked with far greater feeling.

The room suddenly stiffened. The CEO had made his presence known and was walking to the stage. He climbed up and dished out a couple of play punches to one of the other speakers, who moments earlier had revealed how difficult it had been to come out as gay. Presumably the CEO was indicating he was fine with that, but in a way which left no doubt about his own firmly heterosexual standing. He took a microphone and said how wonderful it had been to hear our stories. Aware of his audience, he left it at that, and moved on to say he was fully in support of women at the company, to ensure equality happened at every level. 'But', he said, and you could feel it coming, 'we have to increase those profits first! Then we can start to move everyone up to the same level.'

I looked around and saw several women die inside. I'd heard this kind of thing before from senior executives at big companies:

they're all for equal pay, but the men can't take a hit, so in order for women to gain parity, more money needs to be made. *Keep on working harder, ladies, and we'll see what we can do.* And what it really meant from these guys was, 'I'm not prepared to stick my neck out to change anything, not when my job will be on the line from shareholders – but, tell you what, if there's abundant success I'll sneak in equality under the radar.' The reality for most businesses, of course, is that the demands for ever more profit are never satisfied, there is no 'extra' cash, and so for women the painful crawl uphill continues.

Equality dies on such battlefields every day, and the patriarchy continues. (*'The what? Never heard of it, mate . . .'*)

Thomas Page McBee, author of *Amateur*, and the first trans man to box at Madison Square Garden, told me he couldn't believe how the world changed for him when he became a man. 'It felt like I had a lubricated experience of the world, because I'm also white,' he said.

> Before I had an androgynous gender identity which didn't make sense to people. They didn't know what to do with me. Then suddenly I'd be rolling through a toll booth and have someone say, 'Hey, brother!' That was so odd. And upsetting, I guess: 'Why should I have this? Why can't people treat everyone this way?' The level of privilege is unbelievable.

We'd met in a pirate-themed bookshop in north London where, with his tattoos and sharp-eyed energy, he fitted right in. Trans people are today living proof of the flexibility of gender identity, that it is a complex conversation between genetics, hormones, sexual characteristics, upbringing, life experience and more – and that a person can actively develop their favoured form if they have the courage and support to really go for it. But after Thomas became the man he always wanted to be, he found it brought all kinds of conflict: his 'romantic' vision of masculinity – which included a desire to test himself in the macho world of boxing – was confronted with the reality of the male experience, of assumed superiority and physical threat, where lone women would cross the street at night to avoid him. He went from Other to the Norm, which in certain respects turned out to be tough to take: 'I have the privilege of being able to pass through the world as a man. Because that is where all those privileges come from – it's not from being trans, obviously: it's from people not knowing I'm trans.'

In his book, Thomas addresses his situation by asking questions of himself. Like whether he was sexist. Despite his experience, and despite being a feminist, had he absorbed sexism from the society in which he lives? 'I kept track,' he said, 'and noticed at work I'd interrupt women more than men, speak over women more, answer men's emails quicker. Once I had that data I was able to rethink the way I was acting at work.' He'd make sure female team members were given room to contribute in meetings, and he'd ask for their help with his work; leading the way with small but crucial measures which are still beyond the comprehension of many men. ('Ask for help? I'd rather be fired . . .')

Thomas is now asking men to evaluate their own behaviour, to become conscious of their status and the unconscious ways of going about things that come with it, and work on improving the lives of the people around them. When I asked him what you can do if, despite your best intentions, you're worried you may be considered toxic, he said, 'You probably are!

But that's not because you are failing; it's not because you have failed to become a good man: it's because you live in a culture where you have been taught to behave in a certain way and which you have internalised . . . The solution is not to say, 'Oh, I'm a bad person,' or, 'No way, I never learned that,' because you would be the one person who escaped socialization! It's about understanding the system and seeing where you are – and then you can change it.

The uncomfortable truth for men is that when we look at some of our behaviour over the years, there can be moments of profound shame. Old standard male attitudes and behaviours which were prevalent for generations – casual homophobia, casual misogyny, casual racism – have lingered. What used to be celebrated in male circles – 'Total *lad*! Oi, oi!' etc. – is being called out as symptomatic of a whole system of oppressive behaviour towards Others. Understanding and acknowledging that the world entitles men to get away with a lot of unacceptable behaviour is the first step to addressing this and setting a better example.

To defensively dismiss it, and the very notion of a patriarchy, on the other hand, would be to ignore a tsunami of voices and evidence – and actual crimes.

The 'straight white men first' nature of the system breeds prejudice – also the resulting violence, which comes from a conviction that the victim isn't really human. Being sub-Normal, they are of no consequence, so who cares what you do to them? This contemptuous cruelty is the root of hate crimes, which in the UK since 2012–13 have doubled (race-hate crimes making up 76 per cent); in 2018–19 trans-hate crimes were up 37 per cent on the previous year. The idea of the 'less-than-human' bleeds out everywhere, top to bottom, including the language of 'bumboys' and 'piccaninnies' used by the current Prime Minister, Boris Johnson. The defensive male reflex to reject, in order to prove your own strength, treasures ignorance.

Change, however, is not the prerogative of one type of man, even the most powerful. Years of fighting for equal rights, and the emergence of voices on social media, have, for a new generation, ushered in a world of more complex, diverse experiences. Previously marginalized groups have gained strength and support and the opportunity to force change through protest.

Women, half the population, who all this time have had to battle with being 'the Second Sex', have made headway. One notable shift in power has been the rising status of women in business. In 2017–18 the number of women on FTSE100 boards increased to 29 per cent. While across the FTSE100 only six women held the top position of CEO, these companies have been set targets of leadership roles for women, with the government-backed Hampton-Alexander Review requiring that half of all available appointments to the FTSE350's leadership roles in 2020 need to go to women. The type of leaders who run the world economically is diversifying.

Now, whether this kind of policy-led progression is happening everywhere is another matter. Tokenism is rife. Prejudice runs deep. For all the female and BAME entrepreneurs at the front of PR campaigns, if you're a woman you are far less likely to get venture-capital funding for your company, with only 3 per cent of it attributed to female-led companies, and only 1 per cent to women from a BAME background. Launching a start-up has never been easier, but there is a barrier there for the Other, real *and* psychological. Starting your own business may still be pure fantasy for people reminded daily of their status in society: at the bottom.

The other problem is that even with female faces at the top, the system itself can remain sexist. Of the companies with female

CEOs, does equality run all the way through the business? Do they have flexible working for mums? Do they have equal pay, and if not, are they acting on that now, or merely promising to at some rosier time in the future? A gender- and ethnically diverse Cabinet means little if the government it's part of is still ruling over social inequality; if in the same year, 2019, more money is to be spent on repainting the PM's official plane with a nice Union Jack (£900,000) than on local authority projects to target racism (£219,000).

The facts are that if you are a woman you will earn less, do more housework and be more likely affected by a glass ceiling; and you will be punished for having a child, because all those things will combine to make a return to work economically and socially unviable.

In the companies and countries that have addressed some of the issues, the change has been more beneficial for men, too. It has meant more time spent with children to shoulder some of the care time, and less emphasis on work as the sole index of masculine worth. And workplaces employing women do better: according to a study by the Peterson Institute for International Economics conducted in 91 countries, in companies with more than 30 per cent of women on the board profits go up as much as six percentage points. *See, play-punching CEO types, the two can go together.*

The onus, though, is on men to push for this, not just women, or progress towards equality will stall. This means we have to stop gripping the status quo in panic and start implementing change. At work, this means equal pay for women, yes, but also a profound culture change: diverse appointments, a policy shift in working practices and quashing the notion of 'jobs for the boys'.

The implications are vast – politically, legally, culturally and personally – and comprehending the scope of it may make individual responsibility seem insignificant. You often hear men feel 'paralysed' by the feminist outcry. It's easy to assume someone else will sort out the mess. Well, this is one of those huge issues – like mental health support – where there needs to be structural, political *and* personal change, relentlessly, for a long time, in order to get things done.

Male invisibility is a decision to hide yourself within the masculine assumptions of the day. Female invisibility is to be made invisible as an actual person. Invisible males do all right – indeed, as we've seen, the more invisible you can be in the line-up of other men the better: you are 'classically male', and therefore to be trusted. Invisible men ride the invisible escalator of patriarchy to the top, while invisible women mop the ground floor unnoticed.

Of course, there are men who are born into that top echelon, who wield the true power in the country in an Establishment built on a superiority in the blood. The upper class maintains a hold over government, law and media which still dictates not just the way the country is run but *how a man* should run it. Elite education has acted as the forge for the indomitable character of ruling men.

Nick Duffell is a psychotherapist and author who runs a number of important men's groups in the UK. One of his longest-running is called 'Boarding School Survivors', which provides a safe space for men who have been through elite schools and are still suffering the consequences. We FaceTimed as we paced our respective flats – his adorned with books and leather, mine with cheap plastic toys and abandoned bottles of cleaning fluid – and he gave me his perspective on a system of control based on inequality which has a dysfunctional male psyche at its rapidly beating heart. 'We are providing the worst possible trouble for family life and intimacy,' he told me, mapping out a psychological journey spanning the last centuries,

> by breaking attachments from our early guides and putting boys into strange situations, thinking they're not going to come out with psychological problems.
>
> Under Modernism, the technological force which drove the colonial world created a mass dissociation from empathy and vulnerability – it was a rational project. The only way you could deal with colonies the way they did is to dissociate from a level of feelings, which means you can exploit the planet without any conscience; the same dissociation is at the heart of climate change.
>
> In the Sixties Post-Modernism came along to say, 'You're the naughty parent, and we're the good children', but it wasn't a very effective way to correct things: it was polarizing. Then the corporate world kicked back in with Thatcher and Reagan to say, 'Let's get rid of conscience.' Their neoliberalism said, 'Sod the collective, let's do it for the individual.' The whole neoliberal capitalist project is a continuation of the colonialist project, which you exploit for your own good by splitting off things like vulnerability or femininity or collective for progress-driven individualism. All these things line up to how we train the male psyche.

In this country, the top boarding schools still produce the people who hold the power, and the men who do so have grown up with little knowledge of the Other. 'They don't understand women,' said Nick. 'They find relationships with women difficult, and there's often an unconscious misogyny because mother sent them away. It's always the mother blamed, not the father.' Nick has written extensively on the subject in books like *Wounded Leaders*, suggesting that the Victorian emphasis on rationality that still informs the sensibility of the leading schools directly shapes the way countries are run and the values they hold. 'Trickle-down theory doesn't work with economic prosperity, but it works with attitudes.'

Boarding-school kids are taken away from their attachments and put into institutions, which outside of parental control means their development is peer-driven. As we've seen with Ben and Jamie in previous chapters, when you're left to peer-to-peer education it can lead to difficulties. Nick talked about the theory that we have switched from 'vertical education, from father figures to sons in apprenticeships', to a 'horizontal education'. In such closed, tribal environments a boy's emotional life is neither valued nor exemplified, and, coming off the back of successive generations of fathers schooled in the same tradition, by the time they become adults out in the real world this has a direct impact on how society operates at all levels. 'We elevate people who are very poor on empathy and decision-making,' Nick said.

> Because they don't have their emotions available, they cannot possibly understand vulnerable people – because they were forced to disown all *their* vulnerability from the age of eight. We raise our elite to almost take on psychopathic tendencies. And have an education system based on the same Victorian rationality.

This is not to damn everyone who has been through the public-school system, or to suggest that things aren't changing. Jonny Benjamin told me he had done an event at one of the top schools, at a full school assembly, in which one boy stood up to declare his mental health problems, and received a standing ovation. But look at the dynasties dominating the nation, operating as an elite within the elite, and you can't deny it has been this way for a very long time, and its effects still have a grip on the national psyche. For a large section of the population, however, there is reassurance in it: it feels right that Old Etonians should be in charge, because they fulfil the old ideas of what a leader should be: rational, authoritarian, even cruel. Y'know, *a proper leader!*

With the male need to fight for hegemonic status, these leadership ideals seen in workplaces and institutions everywhere – the 'Man in Charge', 'Boss Material', 'Alpha Male' – have shaped the ideals for men as a whole. The fundamental imperative is a denial of feeling; a suppression of one's humanity. 'We have men out there who don't understand their emotional worlds, are afraid of it,' said Nick,

> which means there's this high suicide rate, and a failure in intimate relationships. We have other extreme cases with our ex-servicemen, who we send out to war and expect them to dissociate from humanity as they suffer violence, then come back and not fall to bits. And then you also have kids at the poorest end of society, often fatherless and completely untrained in men's emotional skills, acting out their lost-ness in this terrible violence. For me the whole thing is about bringing men to engage and retrain themselves, and learn to be less rational and better at emotions. It's missing from all ends of our society. I don't think there's anything more important.

Patriarchy may give men the advantage, but it's the top 1 per cent of men who are really reaping the rewards. For the rest of us, you're in a world which only values a small part of you: the bit that grits its teeth, shuts up and neglects its family to squeeze a few extra pence into the profit margin. Valuing your other characteristics, and exploring your emotions, is a form of rebellion against a system which thrives upon a narrow image of men because it makes us efficient workers. It *is* a rebellion, because it is a struggle against forces who actively seek to maintain this order by stoking up a fevered nostalgia about that imagined era when 'men were men'. As opposed to our current incarnations as, what, gerbils?

Women's movements and organizations are usually forward-thinking, proposing changes that will release women from the burdens of outdated stereotypes. The loudest men's voices, of a certain age anyway, are going the other way, back to a time when men held all the power and were never *questioned* about it. Such men don't want the freedom from prescribed gender roles that women do: they want *more bondage* to the stereotypes: *'The problem with men is they've forgotten how to be James Bond.'* Female aspiration is freedom, male aspiration is control.

Expressed by angry sections of men as a backlash on social media – attacking feminists, 'snowflakes', immigrants, vegans, anyone apparently threatening The Way Things Are – their neurotic anxiety involves a misty-eyed view of a past ruled by 'real' men which is so delusional that even sexual assault is defended, or worse, lauded. One of the ways women are Othered and rendered less than human is by being sexualized. The patriarchal system relies upon the idea of women as objects to be won like trophies, impregnated, then caged in the home – and women should be happy about it too: *'Cheer up, love, it might never happen'; 'It already has, fuckface.'* The world is run on psycho-sexual terms in which women are supposed to be playthings for men, not equals. Yet the oppression of women is also conducted on purely sexual terms.

Much of today's debate about male behaviour has resulted from the #MeToo movement. Most women, it seemed, had a story about harassment or abuse. Most men, it seemed, went quiet. Few were active predators, but most had pangs of guilt. There were some retorts about 'natural urges' and shrugs about 'men being men', but the truth was that men had cultural and social licence to act like this, so did. Even Robin Dunbar, the evolutionary psychologist, was adamant that, despite evolution's pull, such behaviour was not an immutable fact of masculinity, and that men should be 'taught courtesy. It is something we once had, but have now lost.' But try explaining courtesy to your average DM-slider with a holiday album of dick pics: '– and this was in Wales . . . cold day, actually . . . This one's better: Crete last summer. Doesn't he look shiny?'

We exist in a system fed by art history, ancient stories, fairy tales, peer-to-peer learning, and now an ever-accelerating grab-and-go digital culture where girls are there to be picked up by boys like any other commodity. Online, offline, it's all the same. You could say women do the same to men, but there's a difference. Jordan Peterson, the influential author of *12 Rules for Life*, which draws on the Adam and Eve myth, wrote that women have been linked to shame ever since Eve ate an apple and made Adam cover his junk: now they have the power to shame because they can choose their suitors. The theory goes that dog-eat-dog male ambition arises out of the fear of being shamed: you work to make yourself as premium as possible so you don't have to face rejection.

But what this leaves out is that, while women can be choosy, men can insist. Often physically bigger, they don't have to take the female 'no' at face value. It's not that all men do this, it's that we *can*, and it's been an accepted social dynamic that we should. If we're real men, that is.

'Persistence wears down the resistance.'

'Did you give her one?'

'Go on, get in there, son!'

Lad talk clichés, perhaps, but you still hear them everywhere in the drip, drip, drip of daily interaction. Harmless locker-room banter? Hardly. Your role, it is clear, is to be hyper-heterosexual: the most effective way of showing your credentials as a successful man. You perform it, and are celebrated for it. To not abide by this code is to be suspect, gay, weird, an Other.

And none of this is restricted to locker rooms.

Anouszka Tate was in the café on the top floor of Tate Modern. Salvador Dalí stared out from a book on the table, tumescent moustache framing his leer. She was describing her commute:

> I have a ten-minute walk between my house and the station, and I will get a minimum of three insults every single day. And have done for six years. 'Slut.' 'Give us a smile.' It's not just one type of man, either: the other day there was a dad with two five- or six-year-old girls telling me my legs were nice. Of course, if you don't respond to them they say, 'Fucking slut', and if you do then it's an invitation for them to follow you home. Now, I get individually men might see it as just one comment – it may be the first time they've ever said anything to a woman on the street. But it's the twentieth time it's happened to me that day, and the last time I was followed home. You might be an all-right person, but my experience tells me to be hyper-vigilant. Of course it's not all men, but it is all women.

Anouszka, highly expressive and articulate in the way the younger generation – raised on coffee, not White Lightning – seem to be, hosts a podcast called Project Pleasure and has a degree in the history of sex and sexuality. Working at the heart of the Sex Positivity movement, she wants to extinguish the old thinking about sex through better education. 'As boys you are taught that you must go after sex,' she said:

> you have a right to it, and that you are not in control of those urges. This perpetuates rape culture. For women sex is a thing boys will do *to* you; sex education is about damage limitation, how to not get pregnant or an STI, or how not to shame the community. Sex is viewed as a traumatic ordeal. Every person I talk to has to unlearn so much.

One of the means by which such pernicious mindsets are inculcated is the language we use about sex. 'The language for men in heterosexual dynamics is about power and making conquests,' said Anouszka. 'It's not about sex. Rather than it being something for you to enjoy, it's something to show off about to your mates. The fact you've had sex is enough: it doesn't matter whether you actually enjoyed it.' We're back to this requirement to always be proving your manhood to your peers, creating another dissociation whereby it's not about the person you're with, but about yourself, and what it will do to your standing. For Anouszka this shows a lack of basic knowledge: 'Boys need to be taught about female anatomy and consent at school' – but you can't let men off the hook, she says.

> I think a lot of the conversation about men changing behaviour has been about, 'What are the new rules?' The rules are just: be a nice person. You'd hope you're a decent human being, and you shouldn't have to be told that you can't touch a woman. If you're annoyed you have to change your behaviour, you're annoyed because you have been caught out, and can't carry on. I don't think the bar has been lifted so high now – we've put the bar at ground level: *be a decent human being.*

Men are aware of this but often stay disingenuous. We are aware of it, but don't want to admit the scale to ourselves, since we're all implicated in some way. The world we have owned is actually quite frightening to large sections of the population on a daily basis. We're not at war, but a hell of a lot of people have to leave the house as though they're going into battle. Equality in work may be increasing, but equal dynamics in social and sexual relationships are a way off. 'So many conversations I have are about, "Well, we've had female prime ministers, I have a woman CEO,"' said Anouszka, 'but it's not about it being illegal to discriminate on gender. Yes, we're all equal in law, but it doesn't mean that my experience of the world is the same as yours. That's why there's a slight disconnect with men.'

The disconnect is related to the dehumanization. Women are Other, and by association *a bit scary*. For all men's supposed rationality, there is a derangement which occurs around the Other: that hand-wringing neurosis which can manifest in straight abuse. Research by King's College found 33 per cent of women in new senior leadership positions reported experiencing disrespectful or insulting remarks, compared to 13 per cent of men. Women may be on the rise, but the backlash is not simply ideological resistance: troll culture, with death threats and rape threats, aimed at high-profile women – MPs, TV stars, rights campaigners – obliterates adult discourse in favour of degrading attacks.

Disingenuousness is dangerous here. 'Bystander syndrome', the enabling of action by wilful ignorance, endorsement by silence, is an undoubted reality: men watching other men take things a step too far, online and offline. More men need to gain the emotional maturity to step out, when it's necessary, of the conformity of being one of the boys; to shape their surroundings as an active enforcer of respectful behaviour. We don't need a fucking Gillette ad to tell us this. Clearly, there's a lot to deal with, and it can't be left to the women to sort out the mess; for men there has to be a switching on and a stepping up.

Anouszka was keen for one solution to some of these problems to be a positive approach to sex and relationships, in which women can take ownership of their bodies as a basis for their worth in society being recognized. For hetero men, meanwhile, it's about clearing a space for that development and actively supporting it, not feeling threatened by it. 'I think this is a great moment to listen to each other,' said Anouszka.

> If you're a man hoping to be with a woman, listen to the things they are saying about what they want. Many men seem to be sticking to an older masculinity, even though women are saying they prefer this more emotional masculinity. We're ready to embrace you with this new masculinity. It requires a leap of faith by men.

A week later, I was at an Intimacy Jam, making a leap of faith. It was a workshop about non-sexual touching, training you to become more comfortable with intimacy. I hate intimacy. I hate people touching me, other than my kids or my girlfriend, and even then I like some written notice. It seemed to me that such stiffness, such cishet fuckboy anxiety, was linked to control, rationality, cultural expectations about what a man should be, and the broader social structure of Default Male power. Was my fear of intimacy, my emotional immaturity, a barrier reflecting a suspicion of other people's humanity? Well, maybe I could start to fix that here . . .

Bells chimed, and music I'd describe as 'acoustic guitar house' started playing.

'Close your eyes and start moving freely around the room. Feel the music in your feet.'

I kept my eyes half open like my kids do when they're checking I'm still in the room at bedtime. I didn't want to bang into any one of these strangers dancing around the tie-dye rugs in what was turning into the kind of rave I'd usually leap fences to avoid.

'Feel your knees, feel your pelvis – let them move.'

If I had to move my pelvis, I was going to stand still. That was the compromise. So I stood there with my eyes closed, juddering on the spot like a petrol station forecourt sign. *How much longer will this go on?*

'And now you are coming back into yourself. Breathe, and feel yourself in yourself. And now, find a partner for some touching.'

I was wearing a cable-knit jumper, my thickest. Precious woollen armour against all this. A woman was nearby. She looked reluctant to partner with me, but there was no one else within range and it'd be unseemly to walk across to someone else.

'Now show your ugly feelings about yourself with your face and body,' said the facilitator.

The woman started making sick faces and sick noises 6 inches in front of my nose. She had her eyes closed, though, so I could look away to watch the other people in the room. And, boy, were some of them going for it. Full Linda Blair in *The Exorcist*, howling and contorting as though they were controlled by an animatronic crew.

The bells chimed, and I turned back to my partner as she opened her eyes. I nodded encouragingly.

'Now swap: the other one has to show their ugliness.'

I reddened and folded my arms. Quietly I said, *Bleurgh.*

164

My partner blinked at me.

Sorry, I said, *I'm not good at this.*

'It's OK,' she said.

I stared at the floor for a bit. Made another half-hearted *bleurgh* sound then gave up.

The bells chimed.

Oh, God – whatever next?

A minute of touching each other, it turned out. Cue very tentative neutral touching on the arms and shoulders. It was awkward. Very awkward. We were supposed to say 'yes' every few seconds to signal consent to continue. 'Pause' if you're unsure, or 'no' if you want it to stop. Quite honestly, though, we were in an unspoken agreement to keep this vanilla: extra-vanilla cheesecake with vanilla ice cream on top. Once I'd spent a minute kneading my partner's elbows it was her turn to do the same to me. I closed my eyes and flinched at every touch.

I was glad my eyes were shut, given the noises from the rest of the room. My exposure alert had been triggered. The easy sexuality of the other people in the session was making me freeze up. I can't get over myself to simply let go. Earlier, as we had sat on cushions in a circle and shared some of our sexual secrets, I hadn't been able to stop saying things like, 'My cock has always been untrustworthy', and, 'Fatherhood has improved my sex life by removing the reminders of how shit I am at it.' People were sharing deep things about themselves, trying to get a handle on their true natures, and I'd have liked to do the same rather than make jokes, but it wasn't happening. I didn't know if I was too Northern, too old, too square or had too many issues to work through, or if, as a typical Default Male, I was prejudiced against even a whiff of hippy. All of the above, probably.

Come on, Martin – shed this shell. Loosen up, go with it.

The people here were young and comfortable with themselves, it seemed. Fresh-faced, empathetic, good dancers even when the music is shite: it looked like a positive new generation. The facilitators hosting were relaxed, charming, tactile, enviable; I sensed sex for them meant candlelit unifications of the soul, not a way to get rid of a hangover.

After two hours in the room it was as hot as the surface of the sun, but my cable-knit sweater stayed on. As my flesh boiled in the bag of my skin, the Intimacy Jam neared its big finish. We had to split into groups of three, for ten minutes each of solid touching, on the ground, by your two partners. Before I had even begun to process this, people were leaping for their preferred partners like randy frogs, leaving me seemingly alone in the centre of the room, last to be picked for the team, a man's worst nightmare.

Then, as in a dream, I sensed a presence behind me.

I turned slowly to see the two biggest blokes in the session standing there grinning sheepishly. All the women in the room, it appeared, had paired up with each other or the nice young lads with fresh skin, and left the looming older men to it. All three of us were over 6 foot, Viking rejects at the Valhalla orgy. We got settled on some cushions and then had to tell each other where we'd like to be touched. From the earlier discussions we knew we were all heterosexual, and I assumed the other two would find this as awkward as I did. The biggest and hairiest of us went first, but was pretty comfortable with it, to say the least. He said he wanted to be massaged hard on his thighs and his glutes. 'Use your fists,' he ordered.

Right.

166

'And also if one of you could walk on my spine that'd be great.'

I expressed concern about breaking said spine, but he was insistent, and the bells had chimed again so we had to begin.

The big hairy man lay down on his front and put his face in a pillow. The other masseur looked at me and asked if I wanted to be the one to walk on the spine, but I shook my head, eyes wide. I wasn't having a paralysed victim on my conscience to top off this afternoon. However, the other man, built like a judo champion, was game and put one foot, then another, on the centre of the hairy man's back, before walking up and down it confidently like a tightrope walker.

'Euuuurgh,' the hairy man groaned.

For a second I thought he'd died, and wondered if these sex people knew anything about disposing of corpses – surely that was a fetish for someone – but then he made the same noise in a more pleasurable tone, so I got to work. While the judo champion was trekking up the vertebrae I started massaging the hairy man's thighs with my fists. It was all fine until he commanded me to do it harder and harder, until I was punching his legs with everything I had while praying he'd forgotten his glutes request. He raised his head to catch my attention. I pretended not to notice until it was impossible not to catch his eye.

'Play with my hair,' he said.

The next few minutes, as I teased his locks with my fingers, were the longest any human has ever experienced. The hair was not my usual preferred brand: I'm used to women's hair, which generally is looked after so well you feel like you're stroking clouds of silk – not men's hair that's washed on the third Tuesday of every month if that Tuesday was the day after Golden Shower Day at the rugby club.

At last the bell chimed. Every sinew in my body screamed for me to dash to the toilet to scrub my hands to the bone, but the judo champ was after an intense massage too, so what was the point? Again, I was forced to use all my strength to knead at his back, thighs and arms. By now it seemed quite amusing that they had to be so macho about it – what would be wrong with some more tender touching? Would it make us any less hetero? And if it did ... well, so what?

When it came to my turn I made a point of asking for a nice, softer kind of massage on my back, with no fists. *Oh, and don't touch my hands.* They didn't question that one, thankfully.

The men set about me, and I felt palms pressing pleasantly into the layers of fabric around my body. Then, as we entered the last few minutes of the day, the facilitator encouraged us to change position. I rolled over onto my back, glancing at some of the other groups, who had progressed to entanglements I recognized from *The Human Centipede*. The other two men looked at me while I made my mind up about what to do next.

How about a nice cuddle?

They were up for it, so I lay on my back and had both of them rest their heads on my chest while I pulled them in close. I couldn't help but laugh; it was nice, though. As the minutes ticked by and I felt their full weight on me I understood the attraction of men, these big old beasts with their heavy limbs and bear-like breathing patterns. It was quite comforting and –

Wait. Is this hairy guy playing footsie with me?

Yeah. He was.

Politely, respectfully, I withdrew my foot. But his foot approached again, like some dude in a nightclub with too much hair gel on. I shifted position to put some inches between us, and a pillow fell onto my head. I left it there, trying to relax, and decided that if he tried footsie again, I'd just let him: less hassle than creating a scene. We three began breathing together as one, the pillow was still on my head, and I was so hot that my eyeballs were liquifying.

The bells chimed!

It was all over.

I opened my eyes and started to get up, and as I did I realized it wasn't a pillow on my head but the judo champ's hand. One was playing footsie, the other was stroking my hair. I felt like a seventeenth-century debutante who'd been ravished by two randy barons while her mother was in the other room. Affronted, I picked up my skirts and made an exit.

Out on the street, putting on my coat, I headed back to my partner and kids wondering why I was so freaked out. Was it the hippy vibes, or the intimacy as a whole, or the fact that I'd been touched by other men? Was I afraid of being gay? That would be absurd. I have always been relaxed about my sexuality, but was I now, at this stage of my life, so conscious of being a Normal Man that the idea was abhorrent? Was I such a long way from gender flexibility, while calling for it in other men? So what if a man was stroking my hair and another man was playing footsie with me? Let them! Who cares? *Don't be a hypocrite...*

It *was* an Intimacy Jam, and we were touching each other in a safe space. Obviously those men were interested in exploring different aspects of their sexuality: a very positive thing. In alarm I'd slammed that particular door in their faces – but in my defence, I hadn't asked for that kind of touching, had I? I'd set rules, as we were entitled to do, and they'd sneaked in some extras.

169

Well, now . . . so this is what life is like for women. Always an arm sneaking around your shoulder, a foot accidentally brushing yours under the table, an erection pressing into your hip on the dancefloor. Insistence, coming from a sense of a right to do what you want. As though a larger physicality gives licence to do whatever you please.

I walked mindlessly through an estate, the stark tower blocks left for dead, boarded-up shops and rotting furniture abandoned on the pavement.

Surely broadening sexuality would help loosen up the system? If men have a multiple number of masculinities to explore, then they must have multiple sexualities too? All that time wasted on defending the hetero-normative masculinity could be spent on expanding outwards as a human. Learning to relax instead of feeling threatened.

It made perfect sense in theory, but in that moment I had struggled with such exploration. I felt it wasn't merely a consequence of the closing in of an ageing masculinity, but my fear of intimacy rearing its head. Clearly I didn't like strangers touching me, out of an instinctive defence of my hand. Added to this was a disturbing rejection of tenderness: human contact was painful to the cold hardness I'd built around me – and really, hadn't the other men simply been tender? It wasn't as though they'd twizzled my penis around, giggling. No, I'd become accustomed to keeping people at arm's length. Generally I need to know someone for ten years before I can give them sustained eye contact.

All things considered, there are huge psychological barriers for men such as me. Despite my minor Other-ness I, like so many men, am a product of the system. There remains considerable work to be done in daily life beyond theoretical support of changes in masculinity, to throw away the little blue blanket of conformity. Along with a recognition that the way to help men in the future is to make sure boys aren't getting closed down with narrow teachings and falling into the old behavioural traps. Freer expression beyond prescribed social roles starts with what's learned at home: the living rooms of our lands are arenas of hope. Shame the men are working late at the office again and may go for a swift one at the pub after.

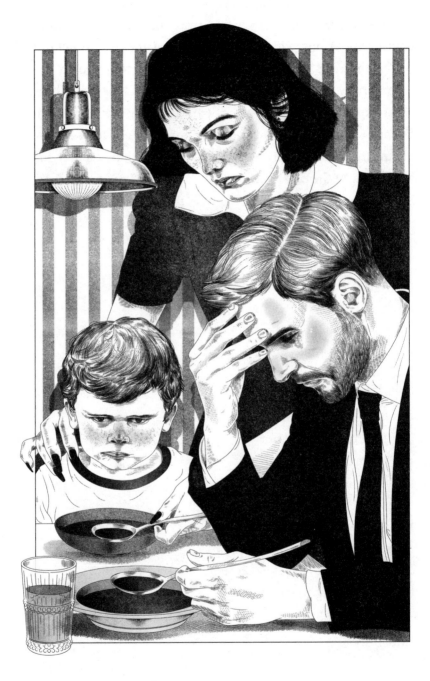

6

You Are the Breadwinner

Home, Fatherhood, Impact

Ambulances were racing by every few minutes. The nearby hospital was turning people away from A&E because there was simply no room; the young were being prioritized for treatment over the elderly. COVID-19 had hit the nation hard, and even though we were finally confined to our homes in lockdown, it was looking like we, as a family, had done it too late.

Our daughter was ill. Marian was ill. I was ill. My son, however, was fine. We didn't know whether or not we had the virus. Marian and I were frightened but hiding it from the children; for days we were simply waiting to see which one of us became worse, who would need to go to hospital – and if this wasn't the virus, we'd be sure to get it there.

In those early days, as the death rate spiked and everything shut down, it was already apparent that this was a national tragedy, a world tragedy, and normal life – going to the shops, having a haircut, meeting friends – suddenly a wild fantasy.

In the second week of lockdown we all recovered, and embarked on the months of isolation together. There was no silver lining here, not with the sheer scale of deaths, but for many people, myself included, it was consoling to think about how life in this country might change when it was all over. The calamitous mishandling by the government was enraging, but I was looking to the people. The unity shown during this crisis, the new connection with neighbours, the revived connections with family and friends, albeit at a distance – all could potentially bring about a new, more caring and empathetic world on the other side. As for men's role in it, I also wondered if more time spent at home could be transformative for them in how they perceived it.

Weeks earlier an innocuous event had taken place, one which had come to seem impossibly quaint: two people in a pub, sat at a table talking, a couple of pints before them and the football on in the background. A tableau of masculinity, you might say: familiar and warm, cheaper than therapy, and with better nuts. Simple pleasures, soon to be lost.

Simon Gunning, the CEO of CALM, was talking to me about the 11 per cent rise in suicide year on year, and why such stats are a barometer for the wellness of a society. The charity had recently launched a new helpline for homeless people, among whom the risk of suicide quadruples:

> We don't know the true figure of suicide amongst homeless people, because the government doesn't give two flying fucks about how a homeless person died. But what we do know is most homeless people are male, and most suicides are male, so you start to think, where is this coming from?

On the screen behind him, Mohammed Salah narrowly missed the target, and the screen cut to fans clutching their faces in anguish. Simon paused, then said,

> When you navigate the causes which go into these massively high-risk groups, there's a familiar story which rings true: somebody

who is male has a traumatic childhood, goes into care, becomes addicted to substances, then goes into prison, comes out and is homeless, and dies by suicide. And it's male, male, male. It has masculinity at the core of it, with other things on top.

We drank in tandem as Simon talked about trying to convince MPs responsible for the justice system to look at the root causes of criminal behaviour, not just punish it. 'And the root cause again and again is masculinity.' As we have seen, men are expected to show strength and power, and when circumstances conspire to prevent such ideals being met, the result can be criminality.

Simon considered his own experiences.

My dad grew up with rationing. I can remember as a kid having one bit of physical contact with my dad, but then the next bit was touching his dead toe. He was dead in his hospital bed – I'd done that thing where you go and say goodbye to your dad on your own – and before I left I touched his toe. And I thought, 'I don't think I've touched you since I was ten.'

You can understand why that is the case: he was a working-class west London man, he did well for himself and ended up managing director of a company and drove a Ford Capri – what more do you want? – but he could not rid himself of that heritage of how men behave. Even though it was clearly very unhelpful to him, and it was definitely unhelpful for me as a child. It was born from this principle after the war, when the bloke next door hasn't got any legs, the other bloke hasn't got an arm, and you can't eat what you want, that you get on with stuff.

People hark back to the past to try to make people feel good about the future. Like 'Make America Great Again', or 'the Spirit of the Blitz'. We are living in the safest time that humanity has ever encountered, this is the finest time to be alive – and yet we almost put notions of masculinity through a regressive filter. To be a real man, you have to use your fists. You have to behave like men did in

the, I don't know, *twelfth century*? Rather than embrace the oppor-
tunities of the freedom of expression that we have now.

I probably tell my son I love him ten times a day. It's part of the
language, it's just part of the way we do things. But a lot of masculine behaviour is mired in the past, and it's mired in a restrictive
nostalgia for the past.

Home is where the heart is, or where the heart is broken early.
The home is the earliest arena for lessons in masculinity, precisely
because the home is not supposed to be a man's place. In the old
messaging, men are supposed to be somehow above the home
space, or at least have a reduced role to play in the emotional world
of those environments; and children absorb these ideas. For us
fathers, the responsibility is huge, but for many years after the war
the development of a child was not particularly seen as the responsibility of a father at all. Work was the man's world, home was the
woman's world. The childhood trauma fuelling so much dysfunctional male behaviour is often due to a disturbing male figure in
the living room, or an empty space where one should be. While a
present father is not a prerequisite for a warm, happy family – as
single mums or all-female or non-binary parents show – when
there is something amiss with the father it can be life-shaping for
a child to a destructive extent. Mothers can be nightmarish figures
too, but men are the focus here, and with men there tends to be
either a desire to perform as the 'Man of the House', or a physical
and emotional absence.

But a father can also be someone with a powerfully positive
impact. Whatever the experience, the impression of masculinity
you received at home as youngsters is hard to shift. Simon, who
was not finishing his drink as fast as me, annoyingly (not that I was
trying to out-man him; I just have severe social problems requiring

alcohol to overcome them, and it was his round), pondered the predicament of all gender relations in this:

> There is something fascinating about the way, when we talk about masculinity, that we just talk to men. But I've got a fifteen-year-old daughter and a thirteen-year-old son, and the masculinity that will be demonstrated around them both will be important to her happiness as well as my son's.

If the world needs to change in the name of equality, fathers have to be engaged at home, for some very practical reasons. In 2019 the organization Promundo released a report called *State of the World's Fathers*, which looked at data on 12,000 men from 11 countries, including the UK. It suggested that, while men were expressing a desire to spend more time with their children, with 93 per cent of British dads saying they'd do 'whatever it takes' to be heavily involved in the early stages of their child's life, only 44 per cent reported taking the full two weeks of paternity leave. It is possible for dads to take advantage of the entirety of parental leave while the mother goes back to work – in fact, since 2016 it's been a lawful right – but less than 1 per cent of dads have taken it up. No-one, basically. Why? A lack of real incentives offered by employers who want men to stay focused on profits, unequal pay – women are paid less, so if one salary has to go in a heterosexual couple, it's likely to be theirs, which also sabotages their chances of earning higher in the future – and cultural taboos, all tying into one another. Plus, well, child rearing looks like hard, messy work – *'This is a man's world, we shouldn't have to be dragged into all that faecal matter.'*

I was sitting with Promundo's Gary Barker and his daughter in a Covent Garden bookshop. He's American (his daughter half-American, half-Brazilian), so they looked as if they'd recently stepped out of a glossy magazine cover, while I, coming in out of the rain, appeared to be something the gutter had just coughed up. Gary's daughter was not really part of the interview, but raised many an eyebrow during the conversation: as a young person at university in the States, she was accustomed to gender roles being at the top of the agenda.

Promundo was launched by Gary after he had been working in Rio de Janeiro in Brazil trying to find alternative life paths for boys from the *favelas* to help them stay out of gangs, an experience which fed into his book *Dying to Be Men*. Former gang members were on the staff of Promundo – the organization was launched with 20 such young men – who worked as peer promoters and co-authors of a programme called Manhood 2.0, which has formed the basis of community education in 30 countries. Nowadays, Promundo works with governments and NGOs around the world, gathering data and educating boys and men to tackle gender-based violence and the regressive masculinity which is often behind it. There may be huge differences in men's situations from country to country, but there are commonalities too, said Gary, and the key ones are men being in control of women, and men being the breadwinners. 'The provider trap,' Gary called it.

> I've done fieldwork from Afghanistan to the Balkans to southern Africa, and that's one thing you do always see. Men can do other stuff, meaning caregiving at home, but we feel we have to be the breadwinners first. Even for men we researched who do a greater than typical amount of fatherhood involvement, or are stay-at-home dads, they still have a gnawing worry about what their children or the world will think of them if they're not also doing some kind of work outside the home.

Men align themselves closely with their jobs. A man is believed to be a person of the working world, which means that their job becomes their identity, and workmates their tribe. If a man loses his job, therefore, it can destroy him. When I lost my previous job, I considered it a judgement on me as a man: not a career blip but a failure as a person. The statistics on male suicide in the UK show it most prevalent in regions of high unemployment, and the 40–60 age bracket most likely to take their own lives. Job loss was no doubt a part of this, feeding into family break-ups and addiction, but more than anything a loss of identity, for anyone raised on the idea that a man must be a breadwinner.

Now, as we saw, men in work are increasingly looking beyond the nine-to-five for validation, and discovering fitness training, extreme sport challenges and adventuring as crucial additions to their lives. Their identities now have new arenas in which to develop.

The idea of spending time at home with a family, on the other hand, still appears a far less sexy option. Sure, there's some famous dads out there giving domesticity a bit of Instagram love if the light's flattering, but statistically, globally, there is a gap when it comes to men seeing the home as 'their place'. And particularly on childcare.

When Promundo's *State of the World's Fathers* report looked at what happened when men did take a more active role at home in caring for children, it discovered the impact can be enormous. If men spent just 45 minutes more a day taking over the unpaid care time – the burden of childcare between parental figures disproportionately undertaken by women in heterosexual households – it would allow more time for women to spend on their careers, and improve the wellbeing of both dads and children. Not even Scandinavia, with its Latte Papas, has achieved equality in childcare work, and in places like Egypt and South-East Asia women do ten times as much of it as men; a man there would be ashamed if he did his fair share, and so would his wife. All over the world those same notions persist, of the control of women, the care–work split and men being the provider.

Gary's response to this is not to censure men, but rather to approach things in a more empowering way: 'Of course we need to call men into greater equality *and* we need to understand and empathize that often this stuff, all these restrictive ideas about manhood, are helping men get through the day and fulfilling what they think the world expects of them,' he said.

> The progress in women's empowerment has been about adding qualities, creating space for women to be all they can and have the right to be, but it hasn't necessarily been the same for men. Men are often still stuck in the box of provider, stoic, steady, and he's lost if he doesn't have that. The new movement in masculinity *is* about adding qualities, not stripping them away. A lot of the time hetero-sexual women want someone who doesn't use violence, of course, and who accepts their freedom, who is a nurturing caregiver, but will also kill bugs and change tyres. It's not about one extreme or the other: it's about the huge overlaps in the middle.

Not ending masculinity, but developing it. Championing men to be a more positive presence. There is huge potential here, indicated by the effects of its opposite on children when a man is not around, or sees his masculinity undermined in this female home world and decides to exert his power with violence.

'A big factor we see which drives violence, particularly intimate partner violence, and other forms as well, is what they witnessed at home,' said Gary,

> Especially for a boy who sees violence of a man against the mother, which happens in up to 40 per cent of households in the countries

we look at. Where that happens they are far more likely, about three times more likely in fact, to use violence against a female partner than a boy who doesn't witness that. It's not destiny; many men witness violence growing up and don't repeat it. Typically, men using violence or very controlling behaviour witnessed something similar, chronically, when growing up.

Gary stressed it was not about making the perpetrator into a victim, nor about stigmatizing men who witnessed violence growing up, but simply coming to

> acknowledge that this is a traumatic experience, and to understand that person as a survivor or witness of violence. And using more subtle ways than campaigns or educational tools which acknowledge that not all men have an equal likelihood of using violence against a female partner. It's about understanding the pathways that make some men violent, rather than putting it on anyone with an XY chromosome.

Promundo's work on 'making masculinity visible' – directly teaching boys about respect, consent and anti-violence, as well as working on worldwide research into masculinity with influential organizations like Unilever – has drawn the WHO and governments into its orbit because it is clear: what happens in a country's homes affects the well-being of a country's people.

For Charlie Webster, exposure to domestic abuse is at the heart of the social problems the UK is dealing with today. I spoke on the phone to this charismatic broadcaster and campaigner from Sheffield, who sits on a Ministry of Justice panel to represent victims of domestic and sexual abuse, and she told me the effects are everywhere:

> We don't change society because we don't look at root causes. Domestic abuse feeds into everything. If we look at homelessness

or knife crime, we do not look at why these things happen – domestic abuse is on a mass scale. With knife crime we demonize young lads, so it means we re-victimize them because we haven't taken the time to understand. And if we don't understand then nothing will change.

Charlie speaks for male and female victims of domestic abuse, she said, and is keen for it not to be a gender war. While girls and women are predominantly the victims, and indeed from 2018 to 2019 there was a 27 per cent increase in women killed by a partner or an ex-partner, a third of domestic abuse victims are boys and men. For male victims of domestic abuse there is a pertinent factor relating to masculinity: the prevalent assumptions about men – that somehow they should be able to shrug it off – lead to them being shamed all over again when they can't. 'Language is so important,' said Charlie,

> because a lot of boys and men are told to 'man up'. In one case I worked on, the police told a man who was suicidal because of his abusive relationship by a woman to 'man up' – that could have killed him. Not because of the abuse, but because of the lack of help, and the language used, that made him feel shame.

Charlie grew up with three brothers in a very troubled home. The trauma was the same for all of them, she says, but often society doesn't see it that way. She talked about visiting a project for young lads who, it seemed to her, would rather be seen as perpetrators of violence than victims.

> We also have a problem with language, when victims are seen as weak. I was the victim of multiple abuse, but I was never weak: I was the strongest young girl – because I survived, and I'm sat here today! So why is it perceived as weak that you're a victim of

something that isn't your fault? That makes the victims feel like it *is* their fault, and plays into the hands of abusers, because abusers *rely* on victims to feel fault, which means they never speak out. There's hundreds of young lads on this project displaying harmful behaviour, every one of whom has been a victim, but they all want to be seen as the hard man.

'Domestic abuse' is the term that Charlie uses, instead of 'domestic violence', as the latter term concentrates on the physical, when psychological abuse is as much of a problem. The law is outdated in this regard, as even if you've been through 30 years of hell the police require an incident of assault or GBH to investigate, so that 30 years has to come down to one assault. 85 per cent of victims of domestic abuse never even come into contact with the police or criminal justice system. To address this taboo Charlie produces a podcast called Undiscussable.

From her perspective, home life and environment are the key factors in male dysfunction, particularly when it comes to young lads getting caught up in street violence.

> They aren't born with it: they are taught it. As a kid I only knew what my environment was: it was normalized to me. How can we expect young people to have a good relationship with the world when they aren't shown a good relationship within their own homes?

Charlie pointed out the relationship between domestic abuse and suicide: how it is a shard of glass spearing many of the most extreme problems:

> The leading cause of homelessness is domestic abuse. Substance and alcohol abuse are really common in young boys brought up in abuse and neglect: they look to drugs and alcohol not as a casual thing but as a way to self-soothe. Why do we never look at why young people

do that? Instead, we treat them as if they're not worth it. The more we show them they're not worth it, the more we emphasize what they've been taught as young kids. Do you know what? When I was a kid, we didn't carry knives, but I was absolutely on the street with an attitude of survival. Anybody – you, me, anybody in government or anybody sat on their high horse – if they were in the same position as these lads, they'd do the same thing.

It is a profound truth about masculinity: that a particular environment dictates its particular form. Environment *is* masculinity: when a hegemonic masculinity pertains, it will take men down a certain path of behaviour. All of us perform according to the world into which we are delivered, and the relationships we witness there. We have to build self-worth and value in men and boys beyond simple basic physical display – and *as well as this* there has to be a wider cultural change in what we value in men. Starting with men's role in the home.

Knowing the power that can be wielded by fathers with devastating consequences means we can also champion behaviour going the other way. Kids *flourish* with supportive fathers: that security and warmth provides a solid wall to cushion you or to bounce off. If a dad can be seen as a carer as well as a protector, and a man capable of displaying emotions without shame, the impact on his children and the mark they subsequently make on the world is enormous. This is where we all step up to contribute, to be accountable for our own actions and set our own example, so that our individual actions contribute positively to the collective.

Charlie left me with this advice for men:

Check yourself. It always starts on an individual level. Are you all right? Are you struggling? Do you feel unsafe and insecure? Start to address it, because those are the things that come out in aggressive ways or in maladaptive behaviours. You don't bully in a place of happiness; you don't act hard because you feel OK about yourself. One of the biggest things we can do is to show vulnerability. It is the most courageous and brave thing, but it's really hard to do. I know how hard it is for men to show vulnerability around your peers, but it's about encouraging that. And if there is bad behaviour, it's about being strong enough to say, 'I'm not having that.'

Out in the woods, on the outskirts of Kent at a secret location known to only a few, there is a very large house with a lot of security cameras and a helicopter landing strip. Inside this house someone was waiting for me who was once described as 'not a nice man, but a kind man'. This was by his wife.

Kev used to be in the SAS, and is now a business guru, a government adviser and an enemy of fools everywhere. He does not like faff. Waffling is right out. Visiting him is like going to an anti-wellness clinic where they don't moisturize your skin but strip it all away. That's not to say it's about macho display: Kev tears away any pretence. I enjoy being with him in an almost perverse way because there is no place for me to hide.

I was visiting a few months before lockdown happened to get drunk and get some things off my chest. That is, when I can get a word in edgeways with a man who may just be the polar opposite of me; anxiety is given short shrift, everything is out in the open. He doesn't give a fuck, as he'd put it. His attitude could well be the result of years of coming to terms with a difficult childhood: growing up in care homes, getting bullied at school, suffering abuse, running away, and acts of violence and theft, which eventually led to him being given a choice by a judge at the age of 16: go to prison or join the army. He chose the latter and focused his frightening IQ on climbing to elite soldier status in the SAS. Since retiring from active service, he's done all right for himself. In fact, he's one of those people who makes you think: what on earth have I been doing with my time? I can't even look at the Mustang in his garage; it's too sickening. But what struck me on this occasion was Kev's openness when it came to his family.

During our 'meeting' in his home bar, decorated with rifles, guns, bullets and other memorabilia – I *think* it's memorabilia, it could be an actual armoury – his wife and kids drifted in and out at various times, and it was noticeable how his manner and his colourful use of English didn't change when he was talking to them. Nothing is restricted here. Feelings are right there in the room, raw and untamed, that lovely messy humanity available, grabbed, shaken about. I asked him how he approached his kids' problems. From what I'd seen, dads' interaction with real-life difficulties, anxieties, relationships issues can be minimal, viewing all this as somehow the mother's role. This is not how Kev sees things working for a functional family, and he has consciously created a safe space in which the family can talk. He saw this as particularly crucial for his young son. 'Boys need to understand their emotions,' he told me

> Every Sunday we have a family debrief. We sit down, we go through everyone's action points: what did you achieve, what are you thankful for, what do you look forward to and what do you aim to fix? What did you fuck up? What made you cry, what made you shout? Everyone has to come up with something.

He followed up with a typically forthright sermon about why dads need to take responsibility for instilling socially conscious values in a new generation of boys.

> Distant male parenting – men not being present in their kids' lives, often through working longer and harder at work, or because they're playing fucking golf – means they haven't been raising their

186

children as they should. If boys have a dad there – and it's not just a dad who can do this, but if there is one – boys need him to teach them not to be a cunt. To not be a bully, to not attack, to resist mob mentality, to treat women with respect and that they don't want to be touched. And then someone needs to explain to boys that it's OK to cry, and to shout.

Engagement with boys to encourage expressiveness, then, is key; to not let them bottle it all up. Although it might increase the decibel levels, at least it prevents that damaging and lonely descent into silence.

The SAS provided a code of living that fed into Kev's family life:

Two words: humility and humour. The ethos of the SAS. Humility in the fact you can have any discussion openly and without hindrance, humour wherein you apply a joke to all. As a family we can joke about everything, and the reason we do that is so we have a very open and frank discussion. If any of my kids have a problem they can come and talk to me. People need to stop making everything so stiff. With kids and the identification of emotions and their own sexuality it's all about communication and humility and humour.

The point is not that we should adopt military codes of honour, but that a code of honour is a useful thing to have. To my mind, it is about creating your own. In a man's heartfelt self-examination, what does he want to be? What effect can he have on society? Who can he help?

Later, with us both in a state of psychedelic intoxication, Kev showed me his collection of dinosaur teeth. He scratched a T. Rex tooth across my arm so I could feel the sharp, serrated edges, then he showed me some arrowheads from the Stone Age. I held one in my palm, thought of Cheddar Man and was almost moved to tears (tears which would have been about 75 per cent proof).

The genius of mankind, I dribbled . . . *the miraculous development of our species . . . it cannot all be without meaning . . .*

When those flints were made, it was not with the intention of one day having something to brag about on Tinder: it was about finding solutions to the problems of the day. Rather than being trapped in the past, isn't the excitement of living about trying to advance humanity in the future? And the excitement, the challenge, for men is to look beyond trying to Be A Man to becoming a Useful Human.

Alex Holmes was on the phone, one of a new breed of young men working to educate the next generation in equality and respect. He's the hugely respected creator of the Anti-Bullying Ambassadors, a scheme in which volunteer pupils are trained to act as visible support for children who are bullied in school – there are now 33,000 working in schools in the UK – and also deputy CEO of the Diana Award, part of the late princess's legacy, established to highlight inspirational young people. 'We really do think young people are best placed to change attitudes and change behaviours,' said Alex of his work there,

> and if you give them the skills and motivation and confidence and knowledge they will really make such a big difference. Because all of the studies are showing you're far more likely to respond to a peer. Young people are able to speak the same language, and don't have authority that a parent or teachers have. If you can instil values in a group of young people they can be a real positive force for change.

While more engaged parenting is vital, peer support can't be dismissed. That's peer support, not peer policing of gender. From Alex's perspective, traditional forms of masculinity play a role in bullying. It means bullied boys are particularly reluctant to seek help because they don't want the shame of being weak (which is where the Ambassadors come in). He has also seen that Othering is a major issue, and the cause of a lot of bullying:

> Definitely boys are quick to pull out what is against the norm. There's that phrase 'no homo': if you say something that has thought or affection you have to quickly cover yourself to say, 'I'm not gay.' There is still that typical nervousness around display, affection or any feelings, and anything that shows you are slightly different. Boys are quite quick to pick up on that and make a big deal out of it. That might be a bit of banter, but it might turn into something more threatening.

Alex says the biggest source of these Othering attitudes, according to the kids he's spoken to, is the home.

> We certainly have stories of families watching TV and dads saying something about the people on it, and it rubbing off on the kids, particularly the younger ones. They don't really understand the context, but are just repeating the father figures, who are also influential with ideas that the way to appear strong and man up is to give as good as you get, which will turn you into a hero. With bullying we will hear from boys that a father figure told them you should fight back. It makes our work difficult when the kid has been told at home that you have my permission to lay a hand on a kid at school and sort them out.

It is the classic cliché of misplaced fathering, merely reinforcing the playground school-of-hard-knocks teaching you that you mustn't be weak, you must man up, that to win you must get physical. Instead, time needs to be spent on, as Alex put it, 'dealing with emotions'.

Giving children perspectives beyond their immediate surroundings can, Alex thinks, be transformative.

> A lot of the schools we visit, many pupils will not have ventured out of a town or city. They're seeing the world as quite small, and seeing the attitude within it as the world. Technology hasn't connected people physically: it has siloed people in echo chambers, and unless you go out of the way to access different viewpoints you're not going to get them.

Which feels like a question of safeguarding: opening up boys to different masculinities, too, for a future where they are not trying to live up to impossible ideals of a restrictive masculinity, but have the belief that they can create their own.

Agency. Individual choice and responsibility. Your life is not only the result of the people in the home you grew up in. At a certain point you can find some agency. When there is shame or trauma in your past, there is often a tendency to move forward and never look back, but it is one of the more remarkable qualities of humans that they *can* leave the past behind, pain behind, and go on to achieve. It can be a life-saving resilience. But if you continue to hide the past away, you can find as you grow older that it manifests itself anyway. Looming at your shoulder, guiding your arm, forcing another repeat showing of the scenes still playing behind your eyes. At some stage you have to deal with it.

Social media can nail your past tweeting indiscretions to the wall, and undermine your attempts to grow as a person, but its overriding appeal is to enable you to edit your own life. This screen self is a surface being, a studied persona to present to the world, a performance for a crowd who will never see you shaking with nerves behind the curtain. This can be, as we've seen, what daily life in the world is like anyway – a performative gender experience – but social media has accelerated this tendency, encouraging a kind of addiction to one's own image, coupled with a nightmarish pressure to desperately maintain it. One fuelled by the sport for others on the platform, of spotting any emerging hypocrisies and flaws in the image and, if necessary, dredging up those old 'deleted' posts as evidence of utter moral corruption deserving a face worse than death: cancellation.

The pressure comes on top of all the news-cycle catastrophes, insistent marketing informed by phone surveillance, old schoolfriends popping up to drag you back into the past, cats doing some cute crap, a celebrity saying something dumb, all of it demanding your attention in an ever-accelerating rush. Holidays are invaded by continual emails and work group apps which serve to make even the most mundane office job as addictive as crystal meth. Existence today is a crazed attempt to simply keep up, in which your deeper problems and desires, your psychological tangles, are easily glossed over.

This all plays well with the male psyche.

A heavy curtain was drawn across my childhood long ago, with a few holes offering a glimpse into a denied past. Giants and dwarfs in the sawdust at Hull Fair, grease and toffee smells, screams of excitement, my dad holding both my hands within one huge hand, blowing warm air onto them. A sweet half-time apple, a flask of soup, then running up and down the empty terraces at Rovers on a Saturday afternoon. Grandma and Grandad waving to us from the field in Cottingham as my sister and mother and I rumble by on the Beverley train (there they stay in my mind's eye, still waving). Hiding behind my mother's legs from strangers, perpetually. Hiding behind the sofa from the reaching aliens on *Doctor Who*. Hiding up a tree in the garden, hot with shame. Carrying a suitcase of toys up the road, running away at four years old, safe in the knowledge my mother would catch me, always escaping but never leaving. Then retreating inward. The teenage years difficult to make out, remaining deep in the shadows. The occasional electrostatic spark of memory flashing images of bedroom anxiety, hours spent in a numb and fearful paralysis, eyes unfocused, a person shut down, while I silently built myself the carapace of an adult male to conceal myself in.

Part of the process of a child growing up is to reject the parent. I for one am dreading that. The main instigator of my reassessment of who I am has been becoming a father; more importantly, being with my children has made my expressions of tenderness, love and vulnerability very easy, natural as anything. Now I find myself dreading my children rejecting me when they get older, and necessarily have to go through a process of suddenly viewing me as an embarrassing man who once wrote about being tender with them in some book.

The trick for any dad in such circumstances is to stick around, to wait, because children can come back from the obscurities of adulthood. My dad did, and I came back. Naturally our relationship mainly took the form of talking about sport in the pub, but slowly, as time passed, we talked about family. About his grandfather, who worked for the landed gentry in these parts, a cap-doffing serf, from what I could gather; given my own nervous deference in the presence of posh people this made sense. And I heard about his dad, my grandfather, a bus conductor in Hull, who my dad discovered had another family in the city, and had been through a divorce back when no-one divorced. Although this was never discussed, it had clearly had an effect on my father:

not trauma exactly, more the idea that there was more to people than meets the eye. Everyone is more complex than you know; it's just they usually don't show it. You can only find out by talking through things with someone. There's a lot to be said for my old enemy: talking.

I decided to go back to Andy's Man Club.

I had it all visualized in my head. I'd sit there in the circle, waiting for the ball to be passed to me, feeling the emotion welling. The facilitator would say, 'Anything to get off your chest?' and I'd find myself clutching the ball. A VHS tape would be inserted into the player in my head, and my whole life would run in fast-forward. Chemicals and hormones would flood my system. The Default Male alarm would be triggered, alerting the masculinity police in my mind who would rush to stop me from talking, only to find it was too late:

Last time I was here, I'd say, *I couldn't talk about what was really bothering me. Now I'm going to . . .*

After a pause in which no-one breathed, I'd slowly, dramatically, hold up my left hand.

My hand is deformed. I have three fingers rather than, well, the usual.

The men would look, but there would be no visible shock, merely a sympathetic interest in what I would say next.

It's not much – lots of people have far, far worse conditions, I'd say with compelling gravitas.

The problem is, I could hide it, just put it in my pocket. Which meant I then did anything I could to remain hidden, to stay silent and invisible, to not run the risk of anyone seeing it. And of course it ate me up, became this huge secret, this corruption inside me. If only I had shared it, dealt with it, then maybe things could have been different. It's OK, really: my life is good, and it's not the hand in itself which pains me – it's the years I wasted suffering in silence about it. That's no-one's fault but my own, but now I'm ready to change.

Then I'd allow one solitary Gregory Peck tear to fall. It would be over. The men would warmly applaud me. I'd be calm at that point, knowing I could finally move on.

I'd replayed this scene so many times in my head that it was as though I'd already gone through with it, which meant I wouldn't actually have to go. Sentimentality can really mess with your head. I'd be in the kitchen weeping at this experience I hadn't had. My own *bravery*. Eventually it became so ridiculous that I knew I had to go back to Andy's Man Club, at least to see what would happen. Would it really play out like that when I talked about my hand in front of a group of other men? I had to find out.

But as I was prepping my trip, the flashes on the news of a coronavirus became blanket coverage of a pandemic. As it spread from China to Europe, the shelves in supermarkets over here began to empty. I too joined the crazed dads hunting for goods as if in a zombie film. None of it seemed real. When Italy went into lockdown with a huge daily death toll it was inconceivable that it could happen here. Later, it was inconceivable that we ever thought we'd magically escape it. I wasn't going to Andy's Man Club. I wasn't going anywhere. Not for a long time.

After a while the numbers of daily dead due to COVID-19 were just that: numbers. From the safety of your home during the national lockdown, if you were lucky to escape being touched by the virus, it became difficult to comprehend that so many people were struggling for their last breaths on ventilators. Eventually things opened up again to the extent that you could go about

194

your day, with the home-schooling, the new body-weight fitness programme, the inexpert gardening, and almost forget the horror. Only now and again, when you read a story of a family who had lost a loved one, or heard that a friend of a friend had died, or when you leaned out of the window to clap for the NHS workers, did you feel the dread of those first couple of weeks . . .

As time went by I had unconsciously gathered around me, I realized, all the things that defined me. My kids, my partner, my books, favourite films, old music. I was connecting more with my parents, and picking up threads with neglected friends. I loved having my son and daughter at home, the schoolwork, the drawing, all the messing about and even the constant mess. I felt myself filling up with life in a way I hadn't in years. Perhaps it was that death seemed all around: you felt compelled to defy it.

I found myself wondering if this period would be a watershed for men. Forced to stay away from work commitments, for the dads especially there might come, after the initial trauma of round-the-clock childcare and cleaning, an unexpected and fulfilling enjoyment. A new ownership of home, founded in a new comprehension of the realities of managing it full-time. No doubt there were lots of dads who did this anyway, but for many more who usually hadn't the time or the inclination, well, it was surely revelatory. Maybe it was a nightmare for many people, but still I wondered if, in the new world beyond this crisis, there was a chance that men would become fully engaged in their home and not want to let go. Perhaps flexi-time would be an option; perhaps a longer parental leave would be negotiated next time; perhaps those 45 minutes each day would be eagerly seized. Perhaps the world could permanently change.

Utopian flights of fancy were common during lockdown. When you were protected from what the world was actually like you were free to project onto the blank slate outside your window. This particular one was punctured when I discovered that lockdown had caused a spike in domestic abuse. In London charges and cautions leapt by 24 per cent within the first month of the crisis, and the Metropolitan Police suggested many more victims were suffering in silence, fearing their arrested partner would lose their job and so plunge the family into further financial difficulty. Not all homes are a home. Some house not only people but also cycles of generational issues, alcohol addiction and psychopaths. Men would be among the victims, of course, but, as ever, most were women. Additionally, lots of working women were reported as saying that they'd been turned into Fifties housewives, because of male partners who wouldn't do any household duties. You had to wonder: what machinations of defensive masculinity were playing out?

Nevertheless I wanted to stay positive, to believe that things could change. The main fight for people is to find something to believe in that can inform a better way to be. At some stage men stopped that search, and it needs to be restarted. The grave awaits somewhere ahead in the dark, possibly closer than we realize – we have to at least try to find some light in the meantime. Wasn't this virus the chance to start?

The people I interviewed during this period were taking stock in some way. The poet Derek Owusu, author of *That Reminds Me*, was at home with his mum, but said his mental health issues had been difficult because his 'coping mechanisms had gone'. His routine used to involve going out to write, but now he couldn't:

> I've never been able to write anything in my house – I always have to go to the South Bank or somewhere like that. I hope when I come out of this sparks will be flying in my mind. I feel like I'm

going to be able to appreciate people a lot more after this. I'm going to talk to a lot more people. The energy is going to be nice.

The boxer Conor Benn, who was talking to me on the same Zoom panel, said he was enjoying having his dad – the former world champion Nigel – staying with him and having his wife working from home. Recognizing the way he'd stripped back to what really mattered to him, he'd also been reflecting that he was an emotional man. 'People think boxers are tough, but I probably cry more than my wife. I'm a very emotional guy. I'm sensitive. You watch me fight and think, "He can't be – but I am."' Mind you, the thing he was most looking forward to once lockdown ended was 'punching another guy in the face'.

I wanted some of that. Not the punching-another-guy-in-the-face bit, but the gathering of strength, the getting back to basics, with a determination to grasp the spark of life. I wanted the experience to be the moment when a new, more expansive me entered the scene. The rage within me. The injustice. The bitterness. Well, it was a dead end I'd banged my head against for most of my life. When, actually, there was an open door right next to me, if only I could let it all go.

My children believed in me. My partner believed in me. I had to believe in myself. Why hide any more?

And my hand? Well, I'd treat it like my kids do. With no sense of shame, but rather constant humour and honesty: 'Daddy, why are your fingers like that? Do they hurt? That one's *really* weird. Don't worry, I can help you.'

It really was no big deal, and it shouldn't ever have been.

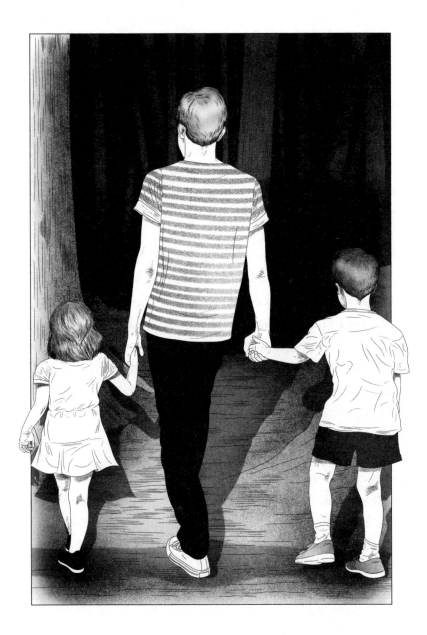

7

You Are a Man

Fear, Insanity, Visibility and the Future

A Real Man does not exist. A true masculinity does not exist. Anyone who says otherwise is either on drugs or works in advertising.

There is not one fixed way for a man to be. If there was, we'd all still be fighting bears in a cave. Instead, civilization arose – and that can't have all been down to women. No, clearly there have been many forms of masculinity in many communities in many different countries at different times in history. Music, art, science, I don't know . . . *beekeeping*: everything shows proof of multitudes of men – humans! – doing so many different things.

Now, there are men today who think we should get back to fighting bears in caves: that this is our genetic destiny as men, and sleeping under a duvet is a betrayal of manhood. These men are usually called Buck. The truth is that we don't have to choose between the bear or the duvet: we can do both, or any variation in between. I for one would be willing to fight a duvet and sleep under a bear, so long as he promised not to play footsie.

It is a question of masculinities, plural. More than one. *Within a single person.* This is what has to be understood alongside the idea of there being many different men: that every one of us has many different men inside.

I can't say how many. It's hard to guess at an average. If I look at myself, I'd say . . . more than four. At least four. But then I have mental health problems due to a mis-managed deformity, so I think I'm more restricted than most.

What I have come to realize, however, is that I have the potential for more expressions of humanity than I am currently exploring. And thus far, I think, a concern with fitting in has limited that exploration. It has restricted my emotional side to something to be done in private, with my girlfriend and children. In the home space I can be daft, goofy, tender, ridiculous, vulnerable, weak, angry, flamboyant and boring, all while the kettle's boiling. When I step out the front door, however, it's like I go through a 3D printer in reverse: I go flat.

It's likely this is the same for everyone; a necessary way of protecting oneself out in the open. For a lot of women, the protection is of a very physical kind. That men are capable of violence, harassment and abuse of every kind is hard to reconcile, but it happens so frequently, against so many targets, that it actually has to be considered part of a normalized male identity. Such behaviour may be attributed to evolutionary impulses, but I'd argue it's a choice made in the belief that this how a man should be. It is taught by authority figures, learned from other men, informed by our culture, and stands on the shoulders of a lot of history. The acceptable face of masculinity is a very unacceptable one.

Brave men are needed. Bravery is about stepping apart from the crowd to act when others have failed to.

Men have to understand this as the world changes around them. The past needs to be let go of because the past is only about safety, about following an old path; meanwhile, the future is going in another direction.

A lot of men in leadership positions are spending their energy holding back that future. The ones who position a cardboard cutout of a strong man in front of them where a human should be. The ones who insist nothing is wrong, and all those on the streets protesting against society's inequality are attention-seeking moaners. Men who have reduced their masculinities down to two: Alpha and Arsehole.

It's suppression. It grips too tight. It smacks of nerves. It's old-school posturing. The future is flexible: it is about communication and diverse experience. Nobody should have to settle for what your family, friends, colleagues, anyone, tells you to be. You have to discover yourself to try to be that wholly original man. It doesn't mean dressing like Blackbeard and doing crack for breakfast – nothing self-consciously 'wild man' – just following your own ideas to enjoy being distinct. Distinction, what a wonderful thing to pursue. Surely a distinct identity is the best route to empathy, the appreciation of other people's distinct identities.

For all to aspire to the same values is lunacy, yet still the Real Man looms; he is comforting. It is frightening to feel you have nothing inside you to cling to, so we want to perform it even if we don't feel it. There is a great deal of fiction out there on What A Man Should Be. A man doesn't cry, a man doesn't kiss another man, a man makes all the money in a household, a man doesn't sit in a passenger seat, a man doesn't wear colourful clothes, a man has pet names for all his tools . . . Boy, does this nonsense wield power. But in their perceived failure to be a man people become dysfunctional. People die by suicide from that shame. And such fictions can be rigorously policed by other men; that they also apply such absurd fictions to women, then police *them* to an even more malevolent degree is truly disturbing (a woman cleans the house, a woman raises children, a woman has to be virtuous, a woman who shows her legs is asking for it, a women shouldn't show her face at all, a woman is sin made flesh).

To be a Real Man, then, is to be a fine actor. You perform the role well, you play your gender according to the dog-eared script.

Men often don't tend to see the relational side of it. The world we grew up in is the only world. When really, if you change your environment or change your tribe, you can change yourself. 'Change yourself' doesn't really mean you change into a completely new person, of course: it means you explore different sides of your personality; you grow. And that's what this is all about: growth. From one masculinity to many.

I think such explorations are actually happening all the time, despite the word not being out. Men can flit between warrior and metrosexual at any moment, go from shopping online for brogues on a train to, in the next second, saving lives in a terror attack. We can change nappies in the morning and parachute out of a plane in the afternoon.

If this can be further explored and idealized, at the expense of an unhinged pursuit of Real Man status, then even the darkest times can be ridden out. Thankfully there are people out there saying this, who can help people escape from the personal hell they've created. People who have broken through from pain to freedom.

Newcastle was preparing for Christmas. The virus wasn't even a rumour, although some say it was around even back then. At the time death on such a mass scale was unthinkable; it was simply one of the averagely miserable days you can rely upon anywhere in England.

I was walking out past the pubs and the kebab shops to the swathe of industrial units circling the city, one of those in-between zones with desolate car parks, sleazy casinos, second-hand car dealerships and abandoned buildings. Another side to a city that you don't see in tourist brochures, but not without its charms.

In front of the Newcastle College, next to the Hong Kong restaurant, on George Street, was the Social. It looked like any trendy new coffee shop, but in fact it was a café and dry bar owned by the Road to Recovery Trust. It offers a place for recovering addicts to work, attend counselling sessions and hang out; for anyone around here looking to break the cycle of addiction it is indispensable. The Social is also famous for its New Year's Eve discos, which 'end with no one fighting, no one falling out, no one arrested. Instead everyone tidies, does the hoovering and goes home in their cars because they are capable of driving.' So said Peter Mitchell, the acting CEO, who was taking me for a tour.

The ground floor was a lively café in a lunchtime buzz, notable for having few noses buried in laptops; the heads were up, in fact, chatting, talking to people across on other tables. Though the venue is open to anyone, it acts as a hub for the addiction problems in the North-East, which has the highest drug and alcohol death rate in England by a considerable margin. 'Over there's the city counsellor for addiction talking to two senior police officers,' nodded Peter, before taking me upstairs to show me the large space for their events and the smaller rooms for 12-step, abstinence-based fellowships. A white board had listed on it: 'Alcoholics Anonymous', 'Narcotics Anonymous', 'Gambling Anonymous', 'Emotions Anonymous' and 'Shopping Anonymous'. Online shopping was the newest major addiction problem, Peter told me. There were other smaller meeting rooms to provide further one-on-one advice, with financial advice a key service. 'Most people in recovery are in massive debt because the addiction has taken everything from them,' Peter said.

> Our service gives them financial inclusion. It helps people get debt relief and budget properly. We have a guy who comes in to appeal benefits decisions for people. In this part of the world there are more than the fair share of economically disadvantaged individuals. We're one of the poorest regions in Europe. The need to escape into addiction is much greater.

Much of the problem when you live in a deprived area, and feel there is no escape except into substances, is that you fall out of the system. In this country the harsh reality is that if you happen to be born into impoverished circumstances, you are deemed less than a person, and the system will keep punishing you with bureaucratic contempt. 'For a lot of people here,' said Peter,

> you haven't got a job, no qualifications, no address, none of the list of things to prove your identity. Passport, or driving licence? Forget it. The best you can hope for is a letter from the DWP [Department for Work and Pensions] – but is that still in date? If you don't have those basic things you're persona non grata in this digital world. You just float about: you're a ball in a pinball machine. Of course, there's a way to escape that: oblivion.

We looked out of the window at the city stretching away. Peter talked about his previous career as a journalist, when he led a team on the regional TV news programme *Look North*, operating with almost total freedom, a thorn in the side of local organizations riddled with corruption or incompetence. His eyes sparkled at the memory. Later he'd keep referring to *once* being successful, but it seemed to me what brought him alive was standing up for people, and he was still doing that: it was simply that, around that core purpose, *he* had changed, and his material trappings were no longer the priority. This can happen when you go to Hell and back.

In TV his life was shaped around hard working, hard drinking and hard men: the culture of Booze Britain, where the line between work and pub gets blurred in the competition to get to the top and stay there. After a couple of knocks Peter became reliant on the drink, swiftly finding himself losing it all and spending his days drinking bottles of vodka in the shadow of a church. The World Health Organization calls addiction a disease, but Peter thought it was a mental condition: an obsession. 'In my case, as an alcoholic, you're either drinking or planning your next drink, and that's not by the shot, that's by the bottle.' Going into recovery was difficult, but the 12 Steps programme of recovery offered by Alcoholic Anonymous worked for him. People are often put off by the religious connotations, but he said it's about creating a God of your own making – 'the universe, nature, or the people in the meeting, who you sometimes also call God: Group Of Drunks' – because you have to let go of your ego and admit you can't rely on yourself. 'All this stuff about alcohol or drugs releasing inhibitions is nonsense,' he said. 'What they mean is, it artificially inflates your own ego – and with men that often comes with aggression. You have to learn humility.'

Humility is something that keeps coming up. One of those core values by means of which you can start pushing masculinity in new directions. Men are supposed to be all-powerful, all-knowing kings of the world, which, when you do find a degree of success, tends to go to your head. The working world, your own tribe, consumerism: all encourage the grandeur of success – of winning! – as the very reason for existence. Humility, though, of letting go of your own ego, has the true power. If your self can become a living hell then it's not simply about building a sexier new one, but being able to let go of the notion entirely. For men, it means dropping the performance of impenetrable control. As Peter pithily observed, 'The cemeteries are full of strong independent men who can just keep going.'

As we've seen, masculinity problems are often political issues, their extremes unveiled by environmental factors, at both the very bottom of society and the very top. 'Lived' masculinity, though, the day-to-day realities of existence, is something which is broad, multifaceted, and can be shifted. If we can celebrate empathy and caring as key qualities for men – and vulnerability as a prized skill – it would allow the development of visible masculinities of a different kind; ones which fight for the well-being of people who need it. More caring and kindness in men will lead to more caring and kindness in society. All it requires is for us to drop the act.

'Virtually everything we do as men is driven by fear,' said Peter.

For me, fear would show as anger. Even when I was successful in my career, people in my work environment would have said, 'He's a bit angry.' But that's just because I was terrified. Terrified of succeeding, of failing, of upsetting people, of not being good enough, of being found out that you're crap. All I'd been doing was acting for thirty years, but never really telling the truth. Never being honest about the way I really felt. Men have a difficulty with that.

Beating fear means confronting it. When I considered how much fear was governing my own attachment to drinking, it scared me. Most of my experiences relied upon it – my very identity, in fact; one shot through with rage. Perhaps the ultimate fear is to lose your identity, no matter how dysfunctional it has become. Actually, to pull apart your identity is a way to transcend it, if you come to realize that what constitutes your identity may have been nailed into place by others, and that the you you thought you were is not really you. 'The answer is inside,' said Peter,

> but in order to get to that point we have to deconstruct ourselves. You grow up, become a man, become irritable, discontented, and you don't know why. You have to deconstruct yourself and reflect, what *am* I about? Battling the herding instinct. We herd into work, we herd to football, herd to the pub, and it's all cobblers. We have to stop and consider who we are, and find out if we're worth saving. I'm sure we'll find out that we are worth it, and possibly valuable to society!

Who are we?

Can we be valuable to society?

I think when we hit a certain point in life one question follows on from the other. If we analyse who we are and save ourselves, we can look outwards at society. Granted, this is the luxury of being a man with the means to consider his position in the world – those that disappear between the tracks are too busy surviving to be able to do so; and in a punishing horizon of pandemic fallout the times are tougher than ever. But those that can ask these questions, must.

What's lacking is morality. This is not a religious or even pious approach, it's about consideration. The pursuit of personal values rather than the perfect capsule wardrobe, and thinking about how they can change our realities.

The belief in yourself as the centre of the world – fuel-injected now by the digital age – can be an empowering thing, but it can also leave you stuck in a roomful of mirrors. With the world in such difficulties it's surely about educating yourself, studying people and figuring out what your wider duties and goals might be. The next move from owning our behaviour is to have a positive impact on the world.

Which brings us back to agency. We know environment – literally location, but also family and friends and the values they hold – will play a role in what an individual chooses to do with his masculine potential. But it is also up to adult men to apply their own feelings and intellect to their lives.

Currently, society's aspirations for men entail a degree of amorality. The top men of society, the moneyed elite, stand for freedom, which includes the freedom to not care; to ruthlessly indulge in every whim power affords. The ultimate male lifestyle fantasy revolves around obscene wealth, dominance over people, private jets, expensive suits, glamorous women, sexy yachts, luxury food, penis-substitute cigars and high-walled private estates for ugly behaviour: this is what success has come to look like. This is pitched as the reward of masculine behaviour, it is the glossy magazine vision, the James Bond dream: the cool, suave, massively minted operator. We aspire to be – and I'm sorry to be colourful about this – cunts. There are no values to it: the achievement is the thing, the end result – if you've achieved that, *you won*, no matter what the human cost, to you or anyone else.

This is why we need a New Aspiration, to do with ethics, depth of character, knowledge, intellect, emotional expansion. You know, the things that make humans happy. Make no mistake, the shifting of male behaviour into new values like this would transform personal relations and bleed out into the way society is run. And for men, developing a mature, more expansive masculinity, which has the confidence to stop worrying about looking like a man and starts to *be* one, is a triumph over fear, over personal trauma, and over the constant anti-life pigeonholing by bosses, trolls, brands, businesses, governments – the whole finger-pointing pigsty that wants to keep you rooted in the shit.

'I think the Taliban are based on a fear of female sexuality.' Mike Snelle was on a roll.

> The patriarchy is based on brute strength and fear of women. Based upon women's sexuality. 'Women want to fuck people? That's scary – she might fuck someone else!' I think the Taliban are based on this: 'We need to make a society where if you fuck someone else we will stone you.' The extremity of that situation tells me it's a deep male thing to be afraid of women. The idea that women have the same desires that we have – that super-freaks men out . . . Why else would you stone a woman to death for infidelity? I think every culture is formed around men being scared of women – *because they're the same!* I could cheat on you, men think, but you could cheat on me, and that's some scary shit.

This is one of those searing truths that can only come after two hours in the pub. The pub was of the genuine old man's type, not the old-man-chic type, down the road from the studio of the Connor Brothers, the cult art duo who have crossed into the mainstream with their subversive paintings and story of the two men themselves, who are not brothers. They were sitting before me in a booth, taking turns to spin theories and articulate their difficulties: Mike, all wiry energy and cutting asides, and James Golding, intense and perceptive, who had come together under the pseudonym of the Connors through the discovery that art might provide a way through their respective mental health problems. We were drinking pre-lockdown, and pre-Newcastle for me; after the interview I'd stay on to drink alone for a couple of hours. But right then, Mike continued with his theory:

> The human instinct is greater than the male or female instinct. People being people. And the things that are gender-related are cultural constructions, and mostly constructed by men, which is why you've got a patriarchy. It suits us. We're stronger than you are, and you're busy having babies, so our shit's more important.

Both of the Brothers consider this, and by extension the society endorsing it, as a trap which brings with it many conflicts. Their success has entailed compromises, the compromises anyone would face as their lives progress.

James came in at this point.

> Isn't that more about the world we live in? Where we're faced with horrific shit all day? Even when you stand up against it you're still part of the system. You're playing a role, aren't you? Even though your subconscious is saying all the time, '*This is shit, this is shit . . .*'

Mike pondered his own mental health experiences, his struggles with suicidal depression. 'Insanity is a perfectly rational response to an insane world,' he said.

> I have been in mental hospitals from time to time, and sometimes I'd say, 'I don't think I'm the mental one here.' We just walked past some homeless people to get here – we're in this absolutely mental world with no compassion and no empathy. Am I really mental,

or am I responding to the fact I'm living in this hostile irrational environment which sets us against ourselves? Maybe I'm not fucking nuts. Maybe I'm sane as *fuck*. And just under this tremendous pressure from an insane society.

With the world becoming ever more divisive and unequal, and led by proudly bone-headed leaders into social and environmental catastrophes, it's no wonder others are echoing this verdict of insanity. The Connors have had plenty of experience with how this can play out for a person entering society. James said he'd always had a problem with his identity, with fitting in, which started in the public-school system. 'I felt different, not as conservative-minded as everyone else,' he said.

> I found myself squeezing into this idea of what it was to be normal. I got a job in the City pretending to be that person. Went into Thomas Pink, bought a shirt and tie: I'm a stockbroker now. Sat at my desk talking about Page Three and football. The guys there were 26, 27, earning three hundred grand a year. They'd smoke crack during the day and heroin at night to sleep. They were robust enough to cope. But for me, having grown up with anxiety, I found heroin took it all away, and I was connected to it immediately. I was trading at my desk in the morning and then in the bog in the afternoon snorting heroin.

Suddenly trapped in a cycle of addiction, it wasn't long before James lost his job, girlfriend, car and house. He was on the streets. 'With no job and no resources it's amazing how you can adapt,' he said. 'On the streets hustling every day, stealing from shops, being involved in violent crime, heists on supermarkets, getting kidnapped, threatened with sexual violence, the antithesis to how I grew up . . . this is cheery, isn't it?'

No, but it was illuminating. For one thing it showed what can happen to a man when he tries to blend in with the lives of the other men around him. It is possible for people to do that and be happy, but if it's not a life you really choose, not something you like, not what you have in your heart, then the consequences – meted out on yourself and others – can be disastrous.

Also on the cheerier side, James didn't die (though he came close), and didn't go to prison (though he came very close). After he was narrowly saved from a five-year stretch his dad helped him get clean, and Mike helped him find employment in the art world. The favour was subsequently returned when Mike fell into suicidal depression and James invited him to move in with him.

That period was the start of the Connor Brothers, where they talked through their respective problems while making art to make each other laugh. The quality and humour of the work won an audience fast and, through a relationship with CALM, they have been able to connect with a lot of other people touched by mental health and addiction problems. James considered a moment.

> The dialogues have been the best bit. I'd never been able to tell someone I shared needles with homeless people in public toilets, and Mike had never talked about wanting to kill himself. When we started sharing the work and people got into it, we became part of a wider group of people who had also had breakdowns. The more popular it's got, the more dialogue we are in with people. It's healthy. Guilt and shame is not talking about things. Now I have the privilege to follow what I want to do, rather than what I think I should do. Breaking down the conformities. I feel like a completely different human being from what I used to be.

As I travelled around the country, chatted on the phone and sat in the pub with all these different people, I was repeatedly shown that the slingshot, the fire lit under all this talk about men changing, in the name of a brighter future for everyone, was mental health. Men everywhere are relating to it.

Simon Gunning of CALM had recounted a story about attending a football tournament organised by FC Not Alone, an organization that brings young footballers together to share mental health matters. 'I did my standing up and talking bit in front of thirty-six teams all sitting in groups on the Astroturf,' he said.

> I was saying, 'We're all coming together doing this: I fully expect to see some broken ankles,' and all that. But then, as I started going into the 'holy shit' suicide numbers, I saw a bloke in one team look at a bloke on the other team, then lean over and shake his hand in solidarity. They didn't know each other! I checked afterwards! The ability for a young bloke to be able to explicitly express solidarity and affection for a stranger in that masculine world was huge.

It feels as if a grassroots revolution is taking hold; a behavioural one. Despite much of the backlash against 'snowflakes' by incensed, red-faced old gits in blazers braying on in the belief they speak for 'the people', the truth is they are on the losing team. 'Average' blokes everywhere are taking a good look at themselves in a way they never used to.

This had been a theme when I'd met up with Ebun Ali, the founder of Mentality Live, a mental health support community predominantly for black men in London, whose message of empowerment and connection has made it a remarkable success story. 'Black men are the hardest target to reach when it comes to mental health,' said Ebun, 'but they're coming to our events, and it is *powerful*.' With their talks and workshops they try to encourage men to see themselves as human when often, she found, they don't. 'I remember I met this guy in finance,' Ebun went on.

> A typical macho man. We had a chat about men, and how their identity is wrapped around what they own, and impressing women. He felt he always had to impress. And I asked him, 'Where's your identity if you took away your car, women, and your job?' And by way of answering he told me his brother had died by suicide a month before. You would never have known he was in mourning . . .

At their events Ebun and her team manage to facilitate a warm environment for truth and tears; it is not a hegemonic space of competing egos, but something else, something new. 'We try to bring that human element,' she said, 'addressing men as human beings, rather than following this ideology of masculinity. The real thing is humanity, and how to deal with difficult emotions, and bring to your consciousness the things that make you happy.'

Ebun noted, as Grayson Perry had, that once you do get men talking, you can't shut them up. They just need a space where they know they're not going to get judged. Look at Andy's Man Club. Around the country it's building. It is about opening up those spaces between individuals too: between close friends. Which of course needs to be a continual dialogue, because, as Ebun pointed out, a mental health problem is not a broken leg which can be wrapped up and healed: it is a constantly evolving maelstrom which needs attention and care. 'Mental health can be a buzzword, when actually it's about identity, trauma and frustration, the real-life human experiences.' She also thought that the question of agency is crucial: encouraging men not only to understand their difficulties but also take responsibility for their own life.

> People think maturity is about having a house or children, but emotional maturity often isn't there. Responsibility is my interpretation of maturity. Life kicks you in the head, but actually you can choose how you react. I think sometimes we have this subconscious awareness of choice, but think we can't change. But we can. Choice is such a powerful thing to bring awareness to.

Responsibility for own your life. It's a transformative idea, one not easily achieved. It is not something that can be imposed from outside. This is why it can be truly life-changing: it must come from men themselves. It can't be faked. And it comes from failure. It comes from mistakes and shame and trauma, which are then reconciled. If a person can admit their problems it can be the start of a process to move on past them.

None of this is to suggest a person must have a breakdown in order to discover who they want to be. Nevertheless, some form of process must be undergone: a new activity, a change of scene, or a period of serious reflection; not waiting until you are fired to embark on a new life; or, for that matter, a virus to come along. I've found that purpose has been a common thread in enabling people to find meaning in life. Finding that thing you love to do, and the inner confidence which comes from growth.

In all of this, risk has to be undertaken, by entering the unknown. It doesn't have to be leaping off a mountain – it can be that more frightening risk: leaping off your own identity. One thing follows another: you have much more likelihood of finding new masculinities and uncovering new talents if you have taken a step away from conventional behaviour. 'I think if men can discover how tenderness is power,' Nick Duffell had said,

> that would make such a large difference. To help men come to terms with vulnerability as normal and human. It's important that when the tender aspect comes out in men they can relate to each other without being afraid of being called a 'sissy'. It just brings so much authority into our contact with each other, and all men have a big role to play in showing this to youngsters. There can be such a knock-on effect in families and society.

Male role models are changing, shifting to those who operate with values and support social causes, and aren't afraid of their emotional sides. Yet changing people's values is a long game; it's taken a hundred years of campaigning to get where we are now with gender equality – with a long way still to go. Change can be a leap followed by a regression, followed by another leap; a wave crashing against the sea wall over and over until it eventually crumbles; as the old world seems to be doing today. And determination is essential, to keep up the fight and bring others with you for the next push.

Which brings up that question again: do men want change?

I think many do. Men do care. They care about other people in society, and I think the message has to go out that they are in a position to shift and cede power for parity with others.

To see them.

The way out of invisibility is to be seen. For me, being seen has always been about love. Along the way I have been lucky enough to be seen by some incredible people in my life, who looked at me and liked what they saw; enough to reach out to help me, push me, be with me. It was remarkable – astonishing! – to feel that love that allowed me to move towards becoming a functioning person. My partner, Marian, saw me in this way and still sees me, every day. I hope that I help her to be seen too. My children make me seen, constantly. If I am not right there, I must be found. Then climbed upon, swung off, questioned, quizzed, prodded, pulled, pulverized – forever undeniably seen. I love it all: it makes me visible, after so long trying to be invisible out of shame.

At home, then, I am human. It is my comfort and joy. But you have to be visible outside too. To set an example for those children and simply for my own sake. For while the process of self-assessment is important for everyone, you have to then show that new, more complete, self to the outside world.

What form that takes is an individual's prerogative. When you have freedom, then you have a choice what to do with it. And yet, I would suggest that for many men like me, the white, hetero, middle-class males who have more freedom than most, there is that job to be done helping those less fortunate to taste the same freedom: allowing others, and particularly Others, to be seen. What did all the men and women I spoke to have in common? A sense of injustice, of righting a wrong, of speaking up for those who can't, of *telling a different story from the one you have been told.*

What man are we supposed to be? Any kind of man we like. That's the point. *Our* choice of man.

The very struggle of a man's life should be to constantly seek to make himself who he wants to be. Life will drag you down in its chaos, repeatedly. The struggle, to the bitter end, is to stay flexible enough for constant renewal, and open enough to explore further possibilities.

For anyone interested in this comes a fundamental choice. Do you accept life as it is, or do you want something more? For yourself and for others. Only the individual, on their own, can answer that.

Lockdown is over, at least for now. We have taken our first day trip in the car as a family, and are walking through the woods. The sunshine is opening the world up and nature is responding, alive around us.

We walk under a canopy of branches flickering with light, throwing Marian into darkness, then illuminating her.

I am carrying my daughter, who is surely in the final year of wanting to be carried. She is certainly heavy, but I won't complain: I'm too busy clinging to the feeling of her arms around my neck, trying to hold it in my memory so I'll never forget it.

My son is running up ahead and then back to me, running and returning as he always does, and as always I'm on the alert for ditches, dogshit, puddles, wolves, anything which might harm him. I bring him closer and walk with my hand on his shoulder for a while.

Even in this moment, I know it is one of respite, not a glorious new dawn. Strife of every variety is coming: economic trouble, job loss, further waves of illness, rising pressures on mental health – the world has been changed by the virus and there is not going to be a utopia. But I am gathering my strength, making plans, drinking less, studying more, trying to learn what I can do to help. I am ready for what's ahead. And it's not here yet. For now, I'll savour this moment: I'm taking it. I'll have this time, these seconds, to keep as mine forever.

I make myself conscious of my hand on my son's shoulder, my left. Ultimately my strange little hand doesn't define me. It has been like a secret burden to carry, but in reality it hasn't stopped me achieving a great deal. Why should it have any kind of hold on me anymore? I am not a victim of it; it's just a part of me.

The sun pours into my eyes. My hand is not a deformity. It is not a deviation from the norm. It is my form, my unique form, following its own design. It is perfect.

I gently squeeze my son's shoulder with it. I feel my son's feelings, and I feel him expand into the future. I want to clear as much of a path as I can before he walks on without me, to learn about the world, learn about himself. Hopefully he'll think of his dad once in a while, and find comfort in knowing I am back here somewhere, always.

My daughter wants to get down, so I gently lower her to the ground. I want her to have a clear path too, free of thorns and low branches, with no limitations set on her boundless joy.

I hold them both for a moment, then let them run along without me.

Acknowledgements

First I'd like to thank Marian for standing by me as I slowly lost my mind at a computer, as well as my last remaining musculature. Your reading and support got me through it. Thanks to my children, too, who coped with the neglect with unfailing good spirits; my son was always ready with a kind word of encouragement, and my daughter simply constructed a toy desk next to mine to at least feel some closeness to me.

Thanks to Jamie Birkett, my editor at Bloomsbury Continuum, for his support of this project, expert advice and belief in me. And to the entire team who have worked on making this book far more than just a bunch of words slapped together.

Also to my agent Charlie Brotherstone, who guided me every step of the way and picked me up out of despair and unhinged paranoia with his wisdom on more than one occasion.

Special thanks to Berta Vallo for creating the wonderful illustrations in this book, but not for scaring me at the cage fighting.

To all the incredible people who I spoke to, heartfelt thanks for giving your time and energy: Ben West, Poorna Bell, Jonny Benjamin MBE, Brendan Stone, Damien Ridge, Robin Dunbar, Jamie and Ben (along with Esther from the DART team at HMP Spring Hill), Simon Gunning, Professor Green, Kitty Nichols, Jason Williamson (and thanks, Claire, for arranging), Fatima Zaman, Jason Fox, Kearnan Myall, Chris Baugh, the Magic Marine, Luke Campbell MBE, Nick Duffell, Emma Sayle from Killing Kittens,

Dr Chris Morriss-Roberts, Joe Gilgun, Cheddar Gorgeous, Tete Bang, Brendan Maher from Movember, Anouszka Tate, Charlie Webster, Kevin Godlington, Alex Holmes, Peter Mitchell, Ebun Ali, Dr Richard Quinton, Derek Owusu, Conor Benn, Gary Barker, Thomas Page McBee and the Connor Brothers – Mike Snelle and James Golding. Thanks also to the organizers of Cage Warriors and the Intimacy Jam.

Particular thanks to Lucy Donoughue from Happiful's I am. I have podcast – sorry again for crying.

Mark Sandford, my fellow *Book of Man* yoke-bearer: special thanks for being on my side throughout all this. It's meant a lot.

Mum and Dad: your love and support means the world to me, as always. And don't worry: despite the evidence in this book, I'm honestly fine . . .

Lastly, I'd like to pay tribute to all the men and boys who have been lost to suicide, and the organizations fighting to prevent this happening on such a scale, with Andy's Man Club and CALM particularly close to my heart. I hope in some way this book makes a useful contribution to that struggle.

Note on the Author

Martin Robinson is the Editor and Founder of *The Book of Man*, a website aiming to support male mental health and wellbeing, and explore new forms of masculinity. He appears regularly on panels, podcasts and radio to discuss his work.

Prior to founding the site, Martin worked in men's and music magazines for 17 years. He lives with his two children and partner in South London.

thebookofman.com / @MartinXRobinson / @thebookofman (IG)

Note on the Type

The text of this book is set in Minion, a digital typeface designed by Robert Slimbach in 1990 for Adobe Systems. The name comes from the traditional naming system for type sizes, in which minion is between nonpareil and brevier. It is inspired by late Renaissance-era type.